W9-BDD-196

ADVANCE PRAISE

"Dr. Anthony Kleinsmith provides a comprehensive overview regarding the supportive science and practical integration of diet, health and medicine with first-milking bovine colostrum. The recipes in the book are creative, yet simple to implement for immediate recovery and health maintenance for your immune system and entire body."

ROBERT SCOTT BELL, D.A. HOM.
Host of the Robert Scott Bell Show

"There is a tremendous need for a book on the power of true colostrum. I have been using first-milking colostrum since 1997 when my radio show started. I have been doing intense resistance training, weightlifting and Hydro-Tone since I was 14 but when I reached my late thirties I stopped seeing any improvement from my workouts. It did not seem to matter how hard and smart I worked out even though I was considered an expert in the field. Two years after I started my radio show, age 49, I started taking colostrum and within a few months I realized I could once again put on lean muscle like I was in my twenties and thirties. Now at 66 I am carrying more muscle and strength than at any time in my life so it goes without saying that I am very, very impressed with first-milking colostrum. But beyond vanity, beyond keeping the body and face youthful, I have seen how powerful it is at keeping me well. Like everyone from time to time I have felt a cold or flu coming on so I simply double or triple my daily dosage of colostrum and it usually goes away quickly or is very short lived. For your own good please find out for yourself how powerful first-milking colostrum is at keeping you young and healthy for years to come."

DANIEL SOLLOWAY PHD, KOKC
Talk Radio AM

"A golden read about 'golden milk,' Dr. Kleinsmith reveals the latest science about the health effects of colostrum for all ages. I especially liked reading about colostrum being the best starter food for growing a healthy microbiome in a baby's gut."

WILLIAM SEARS, M.D.
co-author of The Baby Book

"This is the most informative book on bovine colostrum and will be the go-to manual for anybody who wants to learn more about this anti-aging super food."

MICHAEL LOES, M.D., M.D.(H.)
author of The Healing Response

"Congratulations to Dr. Anthony Kleinsmith for producing the definitive guide to using first-milking colostrum in medicine and health that anybody can understand and whose information can be put to use immediately."

LON JONES, D.O.
author No More Allergies, Asthma or Sinus Infections

"First Milk Diet, is a must-read for anyone who wants to stay alive as long and healthy as possible. Dr. Anthony Kleinsmith has spent a lifetime studying and utilizing the health benefits of first-milking colostrum. He brings this firsthand knowledge to an eminently readable book, that anyone interested in age-defiance will want to read cover-to-cover ASAP."

ROBERT C. MARTIN, D.C., CCN, DACBN, ABAAHP
author of Secret Nerve Cures and host of the nationally syndicated radio health talk program, the Dr. Bob Martin Show

FIRST MILK DIET

YOUR ANTI-AGING SECRET

&

HEALTH PRACTITIONER'S GUIDE

SCIENTIFIC AND MEDICAL RESEARCH
Related To Bovine Colostrum

Its Relationship And Use

IN THE MAINTENANCE

OF

HEALTH

IN HUMANS

WITH SELECTED PUBLISHED ABSTRACTS

By Dr. Anthony Kleinsmith

Copyright© 2016

All rights reserved. No portion of this book may be reproduced or transmitted electronically without authorized consent of the author.

Disclaimer: The author provides the information in this book to acquaint health care professionals and the public with certain health benefits for educational purposes only. The information is derived from a judicious synthesis of traditional and clinical experience and verified by scientific research. It is not intended as a means for patients to self-diagnose and/or self-medicate without the sound judgment and seasoned counsel of a well-informed health care provider. I strongly urge the reader to consult an appropriately educated health care provider before making any changes to health maintenance or therapeutic regimens.

Interior design by Najdan Manic
ISBN 978-0-9968096-0-3
First printing
Printed in the United States
Published by HealthyLivinG Media Group
(800) 959-9797
info@healthylivingmagazine.us

CONTENTS

Foreword *10*

FIRST FOOD

CHAPTER 1—First Milk *13*

CHAPTER 2—Mother's Golden Milk *16*

MEDICINE, FOOD AND HEALTH

CHAPTER 3—Flu Vaccine *22*

Recipe 1—Coconut Chia Pudding *26*

CHAPTER 4—Cancer Prevention *27*

Recipe 2—Protein Rich Vanilla French Toast *30*

CHAPTER 5—One Pill For Over or Under Active Immune System *31*

Recipe 3—Protein Berry Smoothie *41*

CHAPTER 6—Repairing the Leaky Gut *42*

Recipe 4—Café Colostrum *45*

CHAPTER 7—Healthy Blood Sugar *46*

Recipe 5—Almond/Flax Celery Butter *50*

CHAPTER 8—Nighttime Weight Loss Factor *51*

Recipe 6—Orange Lime Vanilla Dream *55*

CHAPTER 9—Dental Health *56*

Recipe 7—Lemon Yogurt Cake *58*

CHAPTER 10—First Milk as Alzheimer's Vaccine *59*

Recipe 8—Café cacao *61*

CHAPTER 11—Heart Health *62*

Recipe 9—Hi Protein Blue Berry Pancakes *64*

CHAPTER 12—Sports Performance *65*

Recipe 10—Lemon Almond Butter *71*

CHAPTER 13—Anti-aging *72*

Recipe 11—Coco Peach Pie *75*

CHAPTER 14—Shopping For Colostrum *76*

Recipe 12—Rich Cherry Chocolate Supreme *82*

COLOSTRUM BACKGROUND

Colostrum background *83*

Chapter References *94*

HEALTH PRACTITIONER'S GUIDE

Scientific and Medical Research related to Bovine Colostrum and

its Relationship and Use in the Maintenance of Health in Humans *99*

RESOURCES

Resources *127*

ABOUT THE AUTHOR

Dr. Anthony Kleinsmith *128*

FOREWORD

I t was my good fortune to serve 12 years in the United States Congress. I left Congress because I came down with Lyme disease from a tick bite I received while fishing at Quantico Marine Base during a Congressional recess.

My Lyme disease was cured by a special colostrum from a cow after conventional treatments were not effective for me. This has started me on a life journey of investigating alternative treatments for disease. My wife and I have formed The National Foundation for Alternative Medicine. We are sending teams around the world to visit alternative clinics and practitioners to see if we can document effectiveness of treatment. We are finding science and treatments that we believe will change the way the world looks at and treats health and disease.

The colostrum treatment that cured my Lyme disease was a special colostrum in which the pregnant cow has been injected with killed spirochetes, the germs that cause Lyme disease. The theory is if the cow had actually been infected with this disease, the unborn calf would contract the disease before it was born, and Mother Nature would cause the colostrum to have ingredients to cure the calf. It worked for me.

As more and more people turn to natural health remedies, as I did, a plethora of scientific studies on all types of health supplements has become available to inform us. One of those items is colostrum.

Colostrum is the nutrient-rich liquid all mother cows impart to their suckling calves when they are born, prior to the release of milk. Its role in nurturing new life, including that of humans (breastfeeding moms also produce colostrum for the first few days after birth), is to impart essential nutrients that boost the health of a newborn as well as to pass on immunities from mother to baby. These immunities protect the newborn's delicate system from the many bacteria and pathogens that exist in their new world.

The same nutrients so important to newborns can also rejuvenate our adult bodies. Once we pass puberty, our bodies gradually produce less of the immune and growth factors that help us fight disease and heal damaged body tissue. The result? Aging. The many nutrients present in bovine colostrum—antibodies, growth hormones, proteins, enzymes, vitamins and minerals—

help restore our bodies to the optimum state of our youth. Research has shown that colostrum supplementation increases energy, stimulates tissue repair, kills bacteria and viruses and optimizes cellular reproduction. Cellular reproduction, as well as an abundance of growth hormone, have direct anti-aging effects.

Though science has been able to isolate some of the compounds found in colostrum, their intake can be questionable. For example, when *The New England Journal of Medicine* reported that growth hormone was the best anti-aging remedy, anti-aging specialists began using it on their patients in earnest. Though recipients reported many anti-aging benefits both external (smoother skin, increased energy and stamina, increased sex drive) and internal (immune system revitalization, organ rejuvenation and less incidence of osteoporosis), it soon became apparent that there were harmful side effects. High blood pressure, the increased growth of unwanted cells in the body (tumors), edema and more turned into reports on the 10 o'clock news as growth hormone therapy came under fire.

Colostrum is a nutritious whole food—the way nature intended it to be. It has been the subject of numerous studies supporting its ability to restore optimum health. We owe a debt of gratitude to Dr. Anthony Kleinsmith for researching this matter and for putting it into this easy to read book, so that people can be aware of and informed of this non-toxic food substance. In a special form it has been of great benefit to me—and, as you will see, when properly prepared, regular colostrum has been of great help to others.

BERKELY BEDELL

Former Congressman Bedell was involved with his friend, Senator Tom Harkin, in the establishment of the Office of Alternative Medicine of the National Institutes of Health. With his friend Senator Tom Daschle he wrote The Access to Medical Treatment Act. He is the founder of The National Foundation for Alternative Medicine.

1

FIRST MILK

My name is Anthony Kleinsmith. I grew up on a small dairy farm in Cache Valley, the main dairy center in Utah where high quality cheeses and other fine milk products are made. By the time I was six years old, my father had me milking cows by hand and, before I was ten, I was routinely doing it morning and night to help out. We were a close family and we all did our share of the chores.

My father always taught me that we had to make sure that newborn calves got enough "first milk" in them to assure that they would develop into healthy cows. He would put the pregnant cow aside and keep an eye on her. As soon as possible after she dropped the calf, he would grab her teats and milk her into a bucket. He would then put some of the "first milk" into a nursing bottle and have me feed it to the calf. That calf would suck on that bottle like there was no tomorrow.

Sometimes my father couldn't be there when the calf dropped and so we didn't get any hand-fed "first milk" into the new calf. We would see the calf suckling on its mother for a little while and then lie down to sleep. Father would watch these calves extra carefully as they grew because they always seemed to be sickly and need extra care and they were never quite as big as the calves that we fed the "first milk."

My father surely didn't know the science behind why getting enough "first milk" into the calf was so important, but he certainly knew the practicality of doing it—the calves that got enough "first milk" were always healthier and became more productive dairy cows and that meant more milk and more profits.

As time progressed, I went to college, eventually earning a doctorate degree in nutrition. My career began in marketing and research for several anti-aging clinics around the world, and I was asked to produce a book on human growth hormone (GH). While working on the book, I found that the synthetic GH used in anti-aging therapies came from a biological source called colostrum. This stirred memories of my youth and I began to put together the relationship between colostrum and the "first milk" that my father considered so important. I went back to the doctors who were running the clinic and showed them what I had found and the response that I received was negative, at best. The person in charge told me that they were aware of some of colostrum's benefits, but that they were only targeting the top three percent of the population with their costly procedures and weren't concerned with anyone else. After that conversation, I quit that line of work to do research on colostrum and its health benefits for humans. I read everything I could get my hands on and l also talked to some of the top scientific professionals in the field. What I found stunned me.

Did you know that in India, where cows are sacred, colostrum is delivered to the home with the milk and is used for medicinal purposes to treat everything from age-related symptoms to the common cold? This practice began several thousand years ago with ayurvedic physicians and sacred healers known as Rishis. In the Scandinavian countries, the birth of a calf is celebrated by the making of a pudding for human consumption from the extra colostrum after the calf is fed. This practice has gone on for centuries and is intended to promote good health. Research conducted in these countries as early as the late 18th century showed the benefits of colostrum on the health and development of cattle and laid the groundwork for the early medicinal use of colostrum by humans. This same ritual was practiced by the early Amish farmers in America.

I found out that there were already a few companies in the United States and other parts of the world producing bovine colostrum-based products and promoting them as dietary supplements for humans. As I read their promotional literature, I found that there were a lot of different things being said about colostrum and its effects and most of the information didn't make sense. Some of the companies were claiming their colostrum was collected from several milking periods after birth of the calf. This contradicted the research from top scientists in the dairy field and it simply didn't fit with what my father had always preached to me about the importance of using the "first milk." Some of the products also made claims about the "advantages" of removing some of the components from the colostrum. This didn't sound right to me either. In my youth, the intact "first milk" was always beneficial to the calf and none of the calves that we ever raised showed any negative effects from getting it. As

I said before, I am a very inquisitive person and the real truth is important to me, so I took my questions to the top scientific professionals in the field. Their answers set me straight and made me a bit upset with the companies that were showering falsehoods on the consumer for the sake of making a profit. I became determined that it was time for me to do something and so I decided to produce and market the finest colostrum available and to bring the truth to the consuming public. My wife and I mortgaged our house and our worldly possessions and our company was born.

We have now been in business for a few years. It has been a real struggle at times for our family but we feel that it has been worth it. We make what sciences says is the best colostrum in the world available to more and more people and are helping them to realize its importance in supporting their own health and well-being. The many letters that we receive from people that it has helped is more gratifying than anything. My father would be proud that we are bringing his "first milk" to the public and that people everywhere are realizing the many anti-aging and health effects he saw on the dairy farm translate well into the human population too.

After getting the company going, I thought that people could lead healthier lives from learning the truth about colostrum and why every anti-aging diet needs first milk. I went back to the scientific professionals who set me straight in the first place and asked them to help me convey the truth to the consuming public. I told them that I did not want any promotional statements or gimmicks that would sell products, but only the true facts in a language that everyone could understand. I also told them that they had to back up what they said with references from qualified scientific periodicals. The following chapters are what I with their help have put together for you. I hope that you will find the truth in them and will learn as much as I did— your health may depend upon it. I've asked Chef Susan Teton, who specializes in bringing whole foods into our diet, to create and share these delicious, nutrition-packed, colostrum-based recipes so you can make this super food part of your daily diet.

2

MOTHER'S GOLDEN MILK

I f you have ever held a newborn in your arms, you have probably been impressed by the helplessness and vulnerability of the child. This baby has just gone from the relative safety of its mother's womb into a world full of harsh sights and sounds, chemicals and germs. It is easy to wonder how something so helpless could ever survive, let alone thrive.

Fortunately, every mammalian species gifts their newborn with a unique first food that is designed to protect and strengthen. This first food is called colostrum. Colostrum is a thick yellowish liquid produced by mothers just before a baby is born. This liquid is especially rich in proteins, antibodies, and other ingredients that protect the baby in its new environment and optimize growth processes as well.

Since every animal's needs are different, every colostrum is different. Regardless of species, when animals and babies get colostrum, they have a much better chance for healthy survival. Numerous studies provide evidence to show that human infants who get colostrum are less prone to infections and are hospitalized less often. These studies even indicate that children who received colostrum as newborns actually perform better academically than those who did not.

Yet, humans do not require colostrum to survive. In most mammals, including humans, many of the critical, biologically active substances are transferred across the placenta, so that they are present in the newborn's bloodstream at the time of birth. These biologically active substances include immunoglobulins, otherwise known as antibodies, and growth factors. For humans and most mammals, colostrum is more of an incredible health bonus than an absolute necessity.

However, cows (bovines) are very different in this regard. Very few of the biologically active substances are transferred to the calf before birth, so the newborn must receive these substances through colostrum during the early hours of life. As a result, bovine colostrum contains more biologically active substances than any other species. These are the same substances found in human and other colostrums but in higher concentration. This means that bovine colostrum can be extraordinarily effective in people too.

The veterinary and dairy industries have capitalized on this information for years. Just ask any farmer what he does when he has a sickly animal or one whose mother is unable to care for it. He gives it bovine colostrum—a practice that has gone on for centuries. Every good dairy farmer and veterinarian has colostrum on hand just in case.

In the last thirty to forty years, our technology has advanced to the point where colostrum can be dried and sealed for use at any time. In this form, people have started taking bovine colostrum as a dietary supplement. It is also being produced in hyperimmune forms to provide vaccinations against some of our most troubling infectious diseases.

I call colostrum an immunotherapeutic medicine of the future. Colostrum is our "first food." It is the perfectly balanced "first meal" that every mammal gives its newborn. It is produced by the mother only a short period of time; yet, it contains numerous compounds to stimulate and support many processes in the body, including activation of the immune system, regeneration and repair of tissues, and growth of *all* types of cells.

The *immune factors* in colostrum provide protection for the newborn against bacteria, toxins, virus and disease.

Many people have been impressed with the potential for "passive immunity" from colostrum—looking for protection from bacteria and viral pathogens. With the regular addition of colostrum to the diet, individuals report a heightened immune response—fewer colds, flu, and allergies. They also notice that when they do catch a cold, they are able to move through it much more easily.

Colostrum's intelligent peptides transmit immune knowledge from the bovine immune system to those who use the first milk as a food; it does so via its immunoglobulin factors. Also known as an antibody, an immunoglobulin is a Y-shape protein the immune system employs to recognize and subdue viruses and bacteria. These augment native intelligence.

Several of the many immune factors contained in colostrum are active in fighting off bacteria and viral pathogens. Lactoferrin is an iron-binding protein with antimicrobial and antiviral activities. Its ability to bind iron keeps many bacterial infections from spreading because the organisms lack the iron necessary in order to replicate. Colostrum's enzymes, including lysozyme and peroxidase, are active in breaking up and hydrolyzing bacteria. Oligo-polysaccharides and glycoconjugates attract and bind to pathogens, preventing them from attaching to host sites in the digestive tract. The above are components that have *active* roles in fighting harmful organisms. Still other immune factors called peptides have regulatory or interactive roles, enhancing or suppressing the production of killer cells, T-cells, interferon and other important substances involved in healthy immune function. Thus, colostrum can help both overactive and depressed immune systems.

Adults who take colostrum do so for a variety of reasons. Many who take it for one specific reason notice positive improvements in other areas of their health. Immune function is just one of the many critical areas of health that decline with age, so do growth factors and nerve protectors. But besides offering replacements for these, enhancing immune function is also one of the main reasons adults take colostrum. Individuals who take colostrum for an extended period of time notice that colds and flu are fewer and further between and that, when they do come, they are not nearly as severe. Many also notice that allergies become less severe or disappear altogether.

Another side effect individuals discover is additional energy. For many, it is almost immediate. It is hard to pinpoint the exact reason why colostrum helps with energy—there are undoubtedly several. Because colostrum helps balance so many functions and contributes to so many processes, it is safe to assume that the energy which would have been expended in these areas is now available for other things. Colostrum also significantly aids the digestive process, which enhances nutrient uptake and utilization. This alone could account for the additional energy many experience.

". . . I have energy that I haven't had in years," says colostrum user Judy D. "I am in my forties but I really feel like I did when I was in my twenties!"

". . . When I began taking colostrum, I initially felt very sick," adds Jill S. "I got a fever and was more tired for a couple of days. Then I got my strength back and I felt more energy than I had felt in three years. The aches and pains subsided and the perpetual sore throat went away."

One user, L. Whetten, found that a long-standing iron deficiency was corrected with colostrum. "I struggled with anemia long before I realized what it was," she says. "I have done many things to try and help my body absorb iron because supplementation alone did not seem to do the trick. Recently, I found out about 'first-milking' colostrum and began taking 1,000 mg a day. Now, eight months later, my blood tests are all in the normal range—finally. My energy level is balanced and I feel good, no more exhausting fatigue. The only change I made was adding colostrum . . . in fact, a lot of days I missed taking my iron. This is the best news I've had in years!" The growth factors in colostrum provide the means for healing and regeneration throughout the entire body. One of the first places colostrum "goes" is to the lining of the intestines. This is where many illnesses actually begin. The lining of the intestines is under constant assault from toxins, microorganisms, refined foods, food preservatives, chemicals and antibiotics. Damage in this area allows pathogens, allergens, toxins and undigested food into the bloodstream where they can cause serious consequences. Growth factors help to seal the lining of the whole digestive tract reducing inflammation and closing the "holes," which result from the above invaders. As a result, ulcers heal, allergies improve, nutrient absorption improves and the line of defense against pathogens returns to more normal function.

Just as the growth factors are able to rejuvenate the thymus gland, they have also been shown to bring new-found vitality and healthy cell growth to heart and lung tissue. These regenerative benefits of these growth factors, which are responsible for the repair of tissues throughout the body, extend to nearly all the structural cells, including skin, muscle, cartilage and bone.

Growth factors are instrumental in promoting rapid healing and repair of damaged tissues in the newborn. They are instrumental in facilitating normal growth and they work with the immune factors to support processes throughout the entire body. For adults and children, these same growth factors are involved in the healing and repair of all types of tissues and organs. With consistent use, they continually regenerate and rebuild the entire body. As with the components of any "food," the growth factors in colostrum typically "go" where they are needed—sealing the lining of the intestinal tract, repairing damaged muscle tissue (including the heart), healing wounds and rebuilding organs and tissues. Growth factors strengthen the gastrointestinal lining to prevent passage of viruses from the gut into the bloodstream. First milk colostrum, it is safe to say, is growth hormone for the masses.

Many of the effects of the growth factors are considered "anti-aging." The youthful "side effects" of taking colostrum include more energy, elevated mood, smoother skin, wrinkle reduction, better digestion, balancing of blood sugar levels and weight loss to name a few.

Dallas S. tells me, "I had an open ulcer on my leg about the size of a silver dollar for four years. Doctors treated me for four months without success. For the next four years I tried everything that came my way—from healing salves and lotions to chlorophyll compounds. Nothing made very much difference, until I found out about colostrum. I began making a thin paste using three or four capsules of colostrum mixed with oxygenated water. I spread this on the wound every morning and evening. At the same time, I began taking eight capsules per day. Within a month there was noticeable improvement and in just two months, all that remained of the original ulcer was a small scab and very pink skin in the area where the ulcer had been."

Arland Reynolds reports, "After having had other heart problems, I was diagnosed with congestive heart failure. I was told that I had an enlarged heart and that there was a certain percentage of it that was actually 'dead.' My doctor told me he had never seen a heart muscle rebuild from that kind of damage. I was told that I would have to severely limit my physical exercise for the rest of my life. I discovered 'first-milking' colostrum . . . and couldn't believe the results. Neither could my doctors. I recently had a number of tests including an echo cardiogram, X-rays and an EKG. After one year of taking colostrum, tests showed that my heart was back to normal size—and now my doctor said that one of the best things I could do was exercise."

For all children—including those not breast fed—colostrum's immune-supporting properties help children in a variety of ways. Often, the combination of synergistic substances in colostrum is enough to boost immunity and clear chronic infections. More often, the components in colostrum contribute to a more rapid recovery and provide support against re-infection.

Children with constant runny noses or chronic infections are some of the ones who can reap the most health dividends. Those who fall victim to every cold that comes along can benefit from the overall support that colostrum provides, strengthening the entire immune system. Most children with these kinds of problems notice that, with continued use, the frequency and intensity of colds and flu diminishes. (The same is true for adults.)

Many children (and adults) with allergies find that symptoms are less intense within several months of taking colostrum. Often, allergies clear up entirely.

Most children who consume colostrum probably do so because their parents are aware of its immune-enhancing benefits. However, colostrum can help children with other difficulties in an unlimited number of ways. Colostrum has so many balancing effects upon the body that taking it can lessen the severity of many conditions and provide early support for super health. Children have a tendency to respond quickly, so the addition of colostrum can often make a dramatic difference. For enhanced favoring there is a form of strawberry colostrum wafers whose taste wins almost all children who try them. (See Resources.)

The Graham family discovered colostrum while searching for something to help their eight-year-old niece who had recently been diagnosed with juvenile diabetes. "At first we got really scared because her blood sugar went up, but we had been told blood sugar levels might fluctuate while the body was finding a new balance, so we kept giving her the colostrum," says her aunt. "Within a short period of time there was marked improvement and insulin levels were reduced. After three months there was no insulin requirement at all—none!"

And the York family notes their two boys with Duchene muscular dystrophy have excelled with colostrum. When the youngest son began walking on his toes, doctors said he was only several months away from undergoing a procedure called "heel cord lengthening" like the older brother had to have. "We decided to give our boys each two capsules of colostrum a day," says J. York. "Several months later, when we visited the doctor again, my son was so much improved that the surgery was not necessary—at least not now. We have continued to give these boys colostrum every day and even the doctors are impressed with their progress. During our latest visit, the doctor asked them to run down the hall and as they did, he watched in amazement. Their coordination was much improved, and my younger son no longer walks on his toes the way he did."

Because of the "wasting" of the muscles with muscular dystrophy, both sons have had trouble getting to the bathroom in time—especially at night and at school where it is not always convenient. Colostrum has practically solved this problem. They no longer have to worry about their embarrassment. "Colostrum has also given back my boys their appetite. They are visibly healthier and we are all happier and encouraged."

However, for most of us, colostrum is a food that keeps our kids healthy and slows down the aging process in our own bodies. The growth and immune factors, combined with colostrum's intelligent peptides that regulate muscle and tissue repair, mean this food consumed regularly is the antidote to the stress of aging. You don't need to be sick to need colostrum. Your body needs colostrum so it won't be sick. The most gratifying part about being involved in bringing first milk to people is what they tell me—how they can't live without it because they feel the difference; how it heals sores and ulcers inside and outside the body; from athletes like Olympian medical winner Winthrop Graham who depend upon it to keep their training consistent and muscles repaired; ordinary people who've used a leptin-rich form for safe weight-loss; hairdressers who've gotten over toxic overload with this diet; it just helps so many people, and that's what I care about and what drives me. I know it will help you and your loved ones. And if you have kids, I urge you to get them on colostrum. Their bodies will thrive with the added immune protection.

MEDICINE, FOOD AND HEALTH

3

FLU VACCINE

Pack child's lunch with food that kills 19 germs

20%	**64.8%**	**25%**
of US population contracts flu annually	of US population doesn't get a flu shot	of immuneglobulins in colostrum

CDC

Each year 5 to 20% of the population gets the flu and more than 200,000 people are hospitalized from complications, the Centers for Disease Control and Prevention reports. Children, even those without severe medical conditions, can die from the flu in as little as three days after symptoms appear, CDC warns. Between 2004 and 2012, flu complications killed 830 children in the US, many of whom were otherwise healthy, in three days or less, according to a report published in Pediatrics. However, we should not be surprised. "Parents don't realize that flu can be fatal," said Dr. Marcelo Laufer, a pediatric infectious diseases specialist at Miami Children's Hospital. Because flu can progress so quickly, prevention is really the best strategy.

Flu shots are the number one method of prevention. But despite advocacy by the CDC, 64.8% of people in the US don't get flu shots.

Maybe we ought to be using colostrum this flu season.

Studies show colostrum works as well as vaccines and synergizes results from the vaccine. A two-month regimen with colostrum in the prevention of flu was compared with anti-influenza vaccination.[1] "After 3 months of follow-up, the number of days with flu was 3 times higher in the non-colostrum subjects," said the researchers.

The efficacy of colostrum an immunomodulator was pitted against anti-flu vaccination.[2] The registry groups included no prevention, vaccination, vaccination + immunomodulators and immunomodulators only. Groups were comparable for age and sex distribution. "The number of episodes registered with the immunnomodulators was significantly lower than those observed in patients using vaccination or no prevention. The average relative costs were significantly lower (2.3 times) in the immunomodulators groups in comparison with the other groups. No problems concerning tolerability or side effects were observed during the study. Compliance was very good. In conclusion, the administration of immunomodulators is very cost effective and appears to be more effective than vaccination to prevent flu."

MAKES ILLNESSES LESS SEVERE

The number one cause of infant mortality today in the developing world is rotavirus. The therapeutic efficacy of bovine colostrum was evaluated in a trial in 75 boys, aged 6 to 24 months, who were infected with rotavirus diarrhea.[3] Diarrhea was reduced by 29 percent among children receiving the colostrum. In 50 percent of the children in the study group, diarrhea stopped by 48 hours, whereas 100 percent of the controls were still suffering from diarrhea. "Colostrum from cows immunized with rotavirus antigen is effective in reducing the duration and severity of childhood diarrhea due to rotavirus."

AFTER ANTIBIOTIC USE

Clostridium difficile is the causative agent of colitis (inflammation of the colon) and diarrhea that occurs following antibiotic intake. A report in the *Journal of Infectious Diseases* demonstrated colostrum is able to neutralize the toxins produced by this bacterium."[4] In fact, use of colostrum is cited by the University of Florida Medical School online medical information service as standard for this bacterium.[5]

FIRST MILK IN LUNCH

Children's immunity responds to nutrition, according to studies. First milk bovine colostrum was also the source of the first polio vaccine. "In 1950, Dr. Albert Sabin, the polio vaccine developer, discovered that colostrum contained antibodies against polio and recommended it for children susceptible to catching polio," reports Zoltan P. Rona, M.D., M.S. in the *American Journal of Natural Medicine*. "In the United States and throughout the world, conventional doctors used it for antibiotic purposes prior to the introduction of sulfa drugs and penicillin."

Colostrum peptides and immunoglobulins conduct immune education courses for the body's white blood cells by delivering antibodies that are already equipped to recognize, attack and neutralize bacteria and viruses that might otherwise slip though the child's defenses.

While colostrum might seem impractical to pack with a child's lunch, it isn't. Strawberry flavored children's lozenges contain first-milking colostrum with growth and immune factors. Lactoferrin attacks bacteria and viruses and is found in saliva, tears and nasal secretions, just where the body's sentries reside. Proline-rich polypeptides regulate the immune sytem's response, making sure it attacks with the right cells and cleans up the toxins later.

Obviously, washing hands, not sending kids to school when they are sick, feeding them immune-strengthening foods such as vegetables and fruits and supplying them with necessary vitamins and minerals is part and parcel of resisting opportunistic pathogens.

HOW TO USE

In cases of flu, take six to eight 500 mg capsules of first milking colostrum daily. Colostrum is a food and you can actually take more or consume by the spoonful as a powder (many people do). For children, give them as many of the strawberry lozenges as they desire—three to five 200 mg lozenges an hour during the acute phase is quite a good dosage. However, the real treasure of colostrum is with prevention. Packing three of the lozenges with kids' lunches will keep them free from the flu and other childhood conditions much more so than without the 700 constituents those super tasty little treats provide.

Bacterial Antibodies Present in Colostrum

Pathogen	Conditions/Symptoms
Bacillus cereus	Food poisoning.
Campylobacter jejun	Gastrointestinal upset.
Candida albicans	Oral and topical thrush.
Escherichia coli	Traveler's diarrhea, urogenital tract infections.
Escherichia coli 0157:H7	Colon tissue death, hemolytic uremic syndrome, renal failure.
Haemonophilus influenzae	Acute respiratory infection, pneumonia, conjunctivitis, types of meningitis.
Helicobacter pylori	Gastrointestinal ulcers, possibly gastrointestinal cancer.
Klebsiella pneumonia	Pneumonia, urinary tract infections, heart and circulatory disease.
Listeria monocytogenes	Meningitis, encephalitis, fetal death, blood poisoning among newborns, the frail and elderly.
Proponibacterium acnes	Acne.
Salmonella enteritidis	Salmonellosis.
Salmonella typhimurium	Food poisoning symptoms.
Staphylococcus aureus	Massive blood and skin infections.
Streptococcus agalactia	Mastitis in dairy animals, urogenital tract infections.
Staphylococcus epidermidis	Wound, mucosal membrane infections.
Streptococcus mutans	Dental cavities, subacute heart infections.
Streptococcus pneumonia	Pneumonia, meningitis, sinusitis.
Streptococcus pyogenes	Massive blood poisoning, accompanied by lesions.
Yersinia enterocolitica	Yersiniosis (diarrhea, arthritis, enteritis, pseudoappendicitis, ileitis, erythema nodosum).

COCONUT CHIA PUDDING

This recipe is so easy and makes for a healthy dessert or snack full of protein. I can hardly keep out of the chocolate version.

1	16 oz can
1 T	Immune-Tree Colostrum6
1	scoop PhytoPro Vanilla
¼ C	chia seeds
1 t	cinnamon or cocoa powder
	splash water
	pinch salt

Raw cocoa nibs, nuts, seeds, raisins, berries and Barlean's Forti-Flax. In a blender, combine the coconut milk and colostrum. Blend softly on low speed. Add the PhytoPro powder slowly while blending. This is just to smooth out the mixture, but not blend it. Add the chia seeds to blend evenly, and pour into serving dishes. Once the mixture is in the serving dishes, carefully place the cinnamon or cocoa powder on top of the mixture and swirl through as it blends. This will make a beautiful dish. You can also blend in the cocoa powder or cinnamon as you blend. As you can see from the pictures, I did this with the cocoa powder. Now all you have to do is refrigerate for a few hours or overnight and the pudding will become firm and creamy.

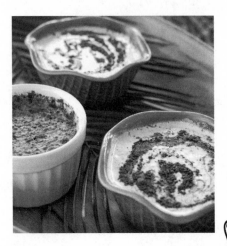

4

CANCER PREVENTION

The immune system normally has a method for eliminating abnormal and cancerous cells. Under normal circumstances, this is accomplished through the efforts of specialized T-lymphocytes called NK (natural killer) cells. Their specific purpose is to seek and destroy cancerous and other abnormal cells. However, NK cells mature in the thymus, which begins to deteriorate after puberty, so the number of NK cells diminishes as we age. This is one of the reasons that cancer is more common among the elderly. A fully functional thymus gland is absolutely vital in maintaining a healthy, balanced immune system that can readily and effectively protect the body against a broad variety of attacks. Cutting down on cancer risk and treating it may involve the potential clinical applications of first milk proteins and peptides, say doctors writing in *Current Medicinal Chemistry*.[6] Luckily, it is also well established that the peptides in bovine colostrum can help to rejuvenate the thymus. Although colostrum supplementation is rarely a cure for those in the advanced stages of cancer, it is highly recommended as a preventive and supportive measure.

Colostrum contains therapeutic proteins and peptides that affect genes and cell signaling. Several colostrum-derived biologics, such as HAMLET (human α-lactalbumin made lethal to tumor cells) and the human recombinant form of lactoferrin, "demonstrated promising results in clinical trials." Lactoferricin peptide analogs are in early clinical development for cancer immunotherapies that educate white blood cells about their enemies. In addition, milk proteins and peptides are well tolerated and many exhibit oral bioavailability; thus they may complement standard therapies to boost overall success in cancer treatments.

CHANGES IN CELL SIGNALING

One of the smoking guns of cancer causation is nuclear factor kappaB (NF-kappaB) signaling. When the genetics are stimulated by NF-kappaB, this increases internal inflammation and increases cancer cells' ability to adhere to tissues and spread.

Human colon cancer HT-29 cells were stimulated with interleukin (IL)-1beta with or without bovine colostrum.[7] By inhibiting NF-kappaB signaling in HT-29 cells, bovine colostrum reduced adhesion molecules and metastasis.

"These data demonstrated that bovine colostrum might protect against [intestinal epithelial cells] inflammation by inhibiting the NF-kappaB pathway," suggesting colostrum has a therapeutic potential for defusing intestinal inflammation and cancer prevention. Additional studies confirm cancer stopping activity.[8] This all makes scientific sense since the gastrointestinal lining has been extensively studied for its rejuvenation effects when subjects are given colostrum (see also Chapter 6).

RADIATION AND CHEMOTHERAPY

During radiation and chemotherapy treatments, the routine use of colostrum can provide substantial support. These treatments, which inhibit growth and metabolic processes, do not discriminate between healthy and cancerous cells and may have undesirable consequences. Bovine colostrum, with its immune and growth factors, restores and maintains metabolic functions while inducing the rebuilding of damaged tissues and promoting the development of new cells. At the very least, it can help to provide cellular energy to fight the disease and the fatigue that naturally accompanies cancer and its treatments.

For chemotherapy and radiation treatments, colostrum should be considered as a front line food; experimentally it "enhances the repair of rat intestinal mucosa damaged by methotrexate" and "ameliorates chemotherapy-induced mucositis."[9] [10] [11] [12] [13]

MULTIPLE PEPTIDES

Until recently, most research has focused on the use of a single peptide for the treatment of a particular condition. There is now increasing evidence, however, administration of a combination of many peptides can result in additive or synergistic activity.

"For example, the coadministration of GH and IGF-I stimulate anabolism and the coadministration of bovine lactoferrin and EGF stimulate the growth of the rat intestinal epithelial cell line...Orally administered colostrum-derived preparations therefore appear to be an attractive therapeutic option because they contain many different growth factors in a formulation that provides inherent protection against proteolytic digestion."

HOW TO USE

If peptides with growth stimulatory or inhibitory effects are to be used, the timing of administration is likely to be critical; growth-arresting factors might protect bone marrow or gut from the damaging effects of chemotherapy if given before chemotherapy, said Dr Raymond Playford and colleagues. "In contrast, growth-stimulating factors might 'rescue' recovery of injured areas if administered after chemotherapy. This latter approach is already being used clinically, e.g., colony-stimulating growth factor is being used to stimulate bone marrow recovery after chemotherapy." [14]

Before using colostrum for complementary cancer therapeutics, please discuss your particular case with your physician.

PROTEIN RICH VANILLA FRENCH TOAST

2	eggs
2	pieces of whole grain bread
¼ C	water
½ +	scoop MHP Paleo Protein, vanilla flavored
2T	Barlean's Forti-Flax
1T	Immune-Tree Colostrum6
1 T	Barlean's Organic Coconut Oil

Low Glycemic–EFA Rich Syrup:

1 T	water
1 t	XyloSweet (xylitol sweetener)
1 t	maple syrup
1 T	Barlean's Flax Oil

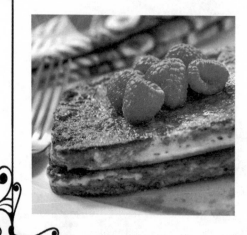

Crack eggs into a bowl and whisk thoroughly. Slowly whisk in Immune-Tree Colostrum6 and MHP Paleo Protein. Note: The mixture will thicken and this will be okay. Add water if needed, but a semi thick mixture will still cook up nicely to provide an extra boost of protein for a breakfast or any meal fit for a day of great energy. Soak both pieces of bread in the mixture for a few minutes, turning over carefully. Warm a skillet over medium heat and melt coconut oil. Place each piece in the skillet and sprinkle the top of each with Barlean's Forti-Flax. Cook until golden brown and then turn, sprinkling the other side with Barlean's Forti-Flax. Remove from heat. Top with syrup (below) and fresh berries.

Whisk all ingredients together for a delicious sweet nutty flavored piece of French toast. Note: It may seem a little runny or thin, but it will soak up fast and make the already delicious vanilla-flavored French toast better than you have ever imagined!

5

ONE PILL

FOR OVER OR UNDER ACTIVE IMMUNE SYSTEM

Among the health challenges women are more likely to face than men are auto-immune and immune-deficiency conditions such as chronic fatigue syndrome, rheumatoid arthritis, systemic lupus erythematosus (SLE or lupus), multiple sclerosis, Addison's disease, asthma, fibromyalgia and Crohn's. Perhaps it is a sign of our toxic polluted environment. Perhaps it is diet and stress, all too sterile environment or all these factors as well as genetics that trips the trigger.

These diseases develop when the immune system attacks various healthy tissues in the body. Multiple sclerosis results when antibodies attack the myelin sheath surrounding nerve tissue, leaving the nerves exposed and vulnerable to damage. Rheumatoid arthritis develops when the joint tissues are attacked. Tennis star Venus Williams was diagnosed with Sjögren's syndrome, an autoimmune disease typically characterized by inflammation in the tear ducts and salivary gland. Doctors are not sure why it focuses on these tissues. Many people will have a very mild form and experience dryness of the eyes and mouth, fatigue, joint pain and myalgias [muscle pain]. Many people will have that and nothing else. But a small proportion of people will go on to have multiorgan system disease that behaves a little more like lupus (another autoimmune disease in which the body's own immune cells start to attack healthy tissues, particularly the joints). A European study found that about 4% of the population may be affected while a study by the Mayo Clinic found a much lower prevalence of around 1%.

It is not clearly understood why the immune system considers the affected tissues to be foreign, but these diseases are a definite indication that the immune system is out of control. Colostrum can help. As we age, our immune system loses its regulatory efficiency as the thymus diminishes in size. Colostrum contains proline-rich peptide (PRP), which has been shown to keep the immune system from over-reacting.

Colostrum provides relief from many of the symptoms associated with these complex medical conditions. For instance, the IGF-1 in colostrum, which directs the metabolic conversion of glucose to glycogen, helps affected individuals overcome the fatigue normally associated with autoimmune diseases. Its growth factors repair and revitalize tissues and organs. Bovine colostrum is widely used by health professionals to treat their patients' cause and symptoms of autoimmune diseases and although only a limited number of diseases are discussed in this section, many other conditions may improve with high quality bovine colostrum supplementation.

Take the case of Dianne M. Tumbers, of Tucson, Arizona. Diane suffered from chronic fatigue syndrome for 14 years when she was first diagnosed with primary immune deficiency.

"I knew that I needed the immunoglobulins [immunologically active proteins] that were in colostrum and I had been trying brand after brand without success," she says. "I was becoming very pessimistic because I knew the immunoglobulins were absolutely necessary for me."

When she tried "first-milking" colostrum, "I was greatly surprised because there was no asthma." She is allergic to milk; the other brands of colostrum had caused both stomach troubles and asthma. "In fact, the 'first-milking' colostrum eventually solved the milk allergy almost entirely," she adds.

"Seven hours after taking those first capsules I stopped getting worse and within several days I was back to 'normal.' The colostrum seemed to help even more than another immunoglobulin product I had used. Also, my digestion, which had been an almost continuous problem for 11 years, is now over 95 percent better than it was. Many supplements and medications give me a rash; colostrum does not and, applied topically, helps heal the skin problems caused by the other substances. I am not yet totally well and I am continuing to take other supplements and medications (although I was able to cut back on some). I know that the colostrum is part of the improvement I am enjoying and I feel very grateful."

One of the reasons true first-milking colostrum has been used so successfully by persons with immune system disorders is that it is a particularly rich source of bioactive immune factors that intuitively act to either rev up or quiet down the immune system. The many immune factors in first-milking colostrum work together to provide valuable immune-support benefits.

First-milking colostrum provides immunoglobulins (A, D, E, G and M), which are some of the most important to immune function. Immunoglobulin G (IgG) neutralizes toxins and microbes in the lymph and circulatory system. Meanwhile, IgM destroys bacteria; IgE and IgD are highly antiviral.

Lactoferrin, also present in first-milking colostrum, is an antiviral, anti-bacterial, anti-inflammatory, iron-binding protein with therapeutic effects in cancer, HIV, cytomegalovirus, herpes, chronic fatigue syndrome, *Candida albicans* and other infections. Lactoferrin helps deprive bacteria of the iron they require to reproduce and releases iron into the red blood cells enhancing oxygenation of tissues. It modulates the release of messenger proteins known as cytokines, and its receptors have been found on most immune cells including lymphocytes, monocytes, macrophages and platelets.

Many drug manufacturers have even tried to isolate and synthesize individual immune factors found in colostrum, including interferon and gamma globulin.

Unfortunately, the drugs doctors prescribe for overactive immune systems are sometimes so powerful that they reduce the immune system to one that is deficient, setting the stage for cancer or infectious disease. Look at the warnings for drugs used with rheumatoid arthritis and elevated infection and cancer risk is one of the hazards of their use.

ONE PILL FOR OPPOSITE CONDITIONS

First-milking colostrum is used for both an underactive or overactive immune system. An overactive one is implicated in autoimmune diseases such as multiple sclerosis, rheumatoid arthritis, lupus, scleroderma, asthma and allergies. An overactive immune system attacks the body's own tissues as if they were an enemy. (An underactive system is implicated in increased risk for infectious conditions, cancer and bacterially related heart disease.)

Colostrum benefits both conditions because it is more correctly thought of as an immune system "regulator."

Also known as colostrinine, PRP is a hormone that regulates the thymus gland, stimulating an underactive immune system or subduing an overactive immune system. In a study published in *Immunology*, it was shown that PRP from colostrum could either stimulate or suppress the immune response.

Proline-rich polypeptide causes the body's immune cells to produce cytokines. Cytokines are proteins that regulate the duration and intensity of the body's immune response. They also are responsible for cell-to-cell communication; boost T-cell activity; and stimulate the body's production of immunoglobulins. Two cytokines induced by PRP include interferon (IFN) and tumor necrosis factor (TNF), particularly IFN-gamma and TNF-alpha.

When it comes to overactive immune system function, PRP "has been demonstrated to improve or eliminate symptomology of both allergies and autoimmune diseases (multiple sclerosis, rheumatoid arthritis, lupus, and myasthenia gravis)," notes Dr. Rona. Proline-rich polypeptide "inhibits the overproduction of lymphocytes and T-cells and reduces the major symptoms of allergies and autoimmune disease: pain, swelling, and inflammation."

SYSTEMIC LUPUS ERYTHEMATOSUS

SLE is a complex chronic autoimmune disease that usually involves several organs. It is one of the most complex and vicious autoimmune diseases and can attack almost any cell in the body. It is much more prevalent in females than males and, in humans, is more common in Asians and African-Americans than Caucasians. Once diagnosed, the disease is usually controlled based upon symptoms, most frequently using corticosteroids. However, it can suddenly fulminate and frequently is terminal based upon end-stage renal disease that results from the formation of immune complexes that block the kidneys. Patients suffer from periodic outbursts of pain associated with inflammation in an organ and are frequently lethargic with low energy due to an associated hemolytic anemia.

The blood of a patient with SLE contains antibodies that attack many normal tissue components. The damage caused by these antibodies includes development of a facial rash, arthritic joint disease, severe hemolytic anemia, heart damage and renal disease. SLE usually follows a slow and irregular course of development during which patients suffer from periodic flare-ups of pain and inflammation. The hemolytic anemia also causes frequent fatigue. Prevalence estimates vary widely, and range as high as 1,500,000 (Lupus Foundation of America). A recent study estimated a prevalence of 161,000 with definite SLE and 322,000 with definite or probable SLE.

Colostrum is rich in thymosins. Thymosin alpha and beta chains are known to regulate the thymus, the seat of the immune system. As we age, the effect of these hormones substantially diminishes and the thymus shrinks. Restoration of thymic control of the immune system is very important in helping to control the immune system of SLE patients.

Susan Rivera has had systemic and discoid lupus for five years and although her symptoms have never been severe enough for her to quit working, the disease was taking its toll on a weekly basis. "The biggest difficulty was the exhaustion," says Susan. "By the time Friday afternoon came around, I was so exhausted that all I could do was fall into bed at the end of the day. I usually spent all day Saturday resting—building up enough energy to do the laundry, clean up the apartment and get ready to do it all over again the next week. I started taking first-milking colostrum on a Saturday morning—just in case I experienced the cleansing reaction I had read about. What little reaction I had only lasted 24 to 36 hours. The following Friday, I stopped off on the way home from work and bought new pots for my houseplants. I went home and repotted all my plants, vacuumed my apartment and made a nice dinner for myself. At nine p.m., I was ready to mop the kitchen floor when I suddenly realized what I had done. It was Friday night and I was full of energy! That was six months ago, but it was the beginning of a whole new pattern in my life," recalls Susan. "In just six months I have made so much progress. I have lost weight, my legs don't burn when I walk, my memory is much better and I don't experience that 'lupus fog' anymore... My head is clear for the first time in years."

Besides the energy, clarity and reduction in pain, the level of infection in her body has also drastically dropped. Since the diagnosis of lupus in 1995, Susan has struggled with upper respiratory problems and ongoing kidney and bladder infections. Her regular visits to urologists have shown sedimentation and ongoing infection for years. However, after several months taking colostrum, her most recent tests showed no sedimentation in the urine and no sign of infection. Her blood tests also showed that she was no longer anemic—another difficulty she had struggled with for a long time. "I take four colostrum capsules twice a day, now, and I feel great!—better than I have felt in five years!"

MULTIPLE SCLEROSIS

One of the most unusual uses of colostrum is with a type developed against the measles. The anti-measles hyperimmune colostrum, which is active against viruses, has shown promise against multiple sclerosis. [15]

The doctors who conducted the study said previous virological and immunological studies have suggested that MS is "triggered by a virus infection." In order to inhibit the growth of measles virus in the patients they obtained a cow colostrum containing anti-measles protein antibodies. This colostrum was orally administered to 15 patients with MS to investigate its effect on the course of the disease for 30 days. Similarly, measles-negative antibody control colostrum was orally administered to 5 patients. "These findings suggest the efficacy of orally administered anti-measles colostrum in improving the condition of MS patients."

Unfortunately, this study has not been followed up on. But it certainly suggests the promising future for a multipurpose vaccine, one that can be consumed orally with fewer side effects, and, depending on what the cows are inoculated with, for so many different conditions.

FIBROMYALGIA

Fibromyalgia is characterized by widespread musculo-skeletal pain, stiffness and fatigue, which are typically more intense in the morning. It is more common in women and quite often there is an accompanying pattern of sleep disturbance. Numerous studies have shown that patients with fibromyalgia have low tissue levels of magnesium even when magnesium is added to the diet. Those with fibromyalgia also have low levels of IGF-1 in their blood.

Both magnesium deficiency and low levels of IGF-1 can be helped by supplementing the diet with high quality bovine colostrum. Many individuals with fibromyalgia report reduced pain and stiffness and they also report better, deeper sleep.

Kathleen Minnion had symptoms of fibromyalgia, which had been getting progressively worse for about two years. "During this time, I also developed a spastic bladder and urinary control had become increasingly difficult. I was very surprised when, within one week after I began to take first-milking colostrum, my bladder problems were noticeably better. Since that first week, I have not had trouble with incontinence. Within three weeks, the knots in my upper arms were gone and the severe muscle spasms had stopped. I was able to walk and exercise with greater ease, which helped even further. After about six months, I had to stop taking colostrum so that doctors could get a clear reading on a series of diagnostic tests. Within days, I went into a 'flare up' and it took colostrum to bring things under control again. Now, I take six colostrum capsules per day. I occasionally experience stiffness—especially when I overdo it, but I am under much greater physical and emotional stress at this point in my life than I was before I began taking colostrum and yet my symptoms are much less. Even during the winter my fibromyalgia is manageable."

The Reverend A. Newman says she was unable to read because she could no longer turn the pages of a book. "I could no longer play the piano or knit or use my fingers for anything. They ached so badly from fibromyalgia. Then I heard about colostrum from a friend. I began taking 20 capsules a day and within nine months I was pain free!!—something I thought would never again be. Now I take one to three capsules each day.... By the way, I am the world's greatest 'tester.' When I am feeling well, I go off the colostrum just to see if it is really working. In about a week or less my hands hurt all over again so much that I cannot hold the cup by its handle. I have done this many times just to see if the colostrum does indeed work. Even the first day after taking colostrum again the pain seems to be alleviated. Thus, after testing my theory many times over the months I am your firmest believer that 'first-milking' colostrum is the best thing that ever happened for my fibromyalgia."

PSORIASIS/ECZEMA

Psoriasis is a chronic, recurring autoimmune skin disease characterized by silver-white scales that form crusty lesions on the elbows, knees, scalp and chest. The disease can also become generalized and involve most of the skin on the body. The skin is often very sensitive to the sun. In the case of psoriasis, antibodies are generated against collagen, the basis of the connective tissue that binds the layers of the skin together.

Eczema and dermatitis are often interchangeable terms that refer to a group of skin conditions also characterized by scaling, flaking and itching. Some forms of eczema are considered to be autoimmune disorders, while others are classified as allergic or hereditary conditions.

It is well-documented that IGF-1 and the associated superfamily of proteins found in colostrum operate in concert with growth hormone in the regeneration and repair of damaged cells. Routine dietary supplementation with high quality bovine colostrum, therefore, is essential for individuals afflicted with such autoimmune diseases in order to assure that sufficient levels of IGF-1 and growth hormone are continuously available in the circulation.

"My grandmother had eczema so badly that she always wore plastic gloves," Mary Fennell says. "I was getting to the point where I thought I would have to do the same. My hands and arms were constantly blistering, splitting, bleeding and weeping—not to mention the continual itching, which was unbearable.

"I had tried a medication called prednisone which worked for a while, but by the time I had finished the first round, the eczema was creeping back—even worse than before. I started taking first-milking colostrum and within a week I noticed a profound difference. My hands began to heal. Within a month, there were no more blisters and my hands had new pink skin everywhere.

I still have a bit of trouble around my ring finger and if I don't take my afternoon dose of colostrum it begins itching by the end of the day. If I go more than a day or two the whole thing starts up again."

Colostrum can have a marked effect on many skin conditions. People notice that the overall look and feel of their skin improves shortly after they begin making colostrum part of their daily smoothies and other recipes.

RHEUMATOID ARTHRITIS

Arthritis is an inflammation of a joint. It can occur in one or more joints of the body and is usually a long-term condition that can progressively disable the individual. Rheumatoid arthritis is by far the most serious, painful and crippling form of arthritis. It can disable an affected individual.

Besides the attack on joints with an associated severe inflammation, it may also affect the surrounding connective tissues and can cause fever, weakness, fatigue and deformity. Individuals with various forms of arthritis, including rheumatoid arthritis, can usually benefit from routine dietary supplementation with high quality bovine colostrum. As with other autoimmune diseases, rheumatoid arthritis represents an immune system that is out of control and the best way to put things back into phase naturally is through routine dietary supplementation with a high quality first milking colostrum. It contains a) specific hormones, the alpha and beta chains of thymosin, that are known to regulate the functions of the thymus; and b) proline-rich peptide that has been shown to keep the immune system under control. Relief from pain, stiffness and fatigue are some of the common benefits. Individuals with arthritis who take colostrum report that they experience much less pain, stiffness and fatigue than before.

"Some 25 years ago I was diagnosed with rheumatoid arthritis and more recently with fibromyalgia," writes Renee Petersen. "Consequently, I have experienced more than my share of aches and pains. But even more debilitating than the pain and stiffness has been the lack of energy. If I wanted to do anything I almost had to build up the energy for several days beforehand and then rest for an equal amount of time afterward—just to be able to do simple things like go shopping. I felt I could live with the aches and pains but I just wanted to have some energy again. One morning about a week after I began taking colostrum, I woke up and I actually felt human. I couldn't believe the difference. Ever since then I have been able to do the things I used to do without that excessive tired feeling all the time. When you feel good, life is so different, and I am happy to feel really good; it surprised me. I worked all day, walked a mile and a half and when I returned home I was even more surprised that I still had plenty of energy. I cleaned my oven and the refrigerator. I swept the floor—then I remembered what I had been told about colostrum and energy. I had given up ever having energy again—but it has been like this ever since that day. I am now taking six capsules per day, and I have the energy to work and to take care of my home too. I'm even walking two miles every day. It's great to feel this good again."

HIV

Take colostrum to give the body additional immunoglobulin-mediated resistance to the human immunodeficiency virus or HIV, linked with Acquired Immunodeficiency Syndrome—that from research reports starting with the August 2012 issue of *Antimicrobial Agents and Chemotherapeutics*.[16]

HIV research from the Department of Microbiology and Immunology, University of Melbourne, Parkville, Victoria, Australia shows that bovine colostrum (first milk) contains very high concentrations of immunoglobulin G (IgG) that kill HIV. "Colostrum-derived anti-HIV antibodies offer a cost-effective option for preparing the substantial quantities of broadly neutralizing antibodies that would be needed in a low-cost topical combination HIV-1 microbicide."

The team says that bovine IgG binds to Fcγ-receptors (FcγRs) on human neutrophils, monocytes and NK cells in a dose-dependent manner—and bovine anti-HIV colostrum IgGs have "robust HIV-1-specific ADCC activity and therefore offer a useful source of antibodies able to provide a rapid and potent response against HIV-1 infection." This could assist the development of novel Ab-mediated approaches for prevention of HIV-1 transmission.

At the Human Vaccine Institute, Duke University Medical Center, Durham, North Carolina, it was found that HIV-specific, functional antibody responses are present in human colostrum and represent two of the first mucosally derived anti-HIV antibodies yet to be reported.

And in December 2011, in the *Indian Journal of Gastroenterology the* Department of Public Health, Gulu University Faculty of Medicine, Gulu, Uganda, reported that HIV-associated diarrhea occurs in nearly all patients with AIDS in the developing countries.[17] Diarrhea is caused by the HIV-related immune dysfunction and is pivotal in the decrease of the helper T-cell population. Enteric pathogens in HIV-associated diarrhea are, for example, cryptosporidium, amoeba and campylobacter species.

An earlier uncontrolled study showed that a nutritional product made from bovine colostrum alleviates HIV-associated diarrhea. The doctors performed a randomized single-blind controlled trial involving the addition of colostrum-based supplement to standard anti-diarrhea treatment in HIV/AIDS patients with diarrhea.[18] Eighty-seven adult patients with HIV-associated diarrhea were recruited at Gulu Hospital and four community clinics in Northern Uganda. Forty-five patients were randomized to receive 50 grams of colostrum-based supplement twice a day for 4 weeks in addition to standard anti-diarrhea treatment.[19]

Expected bathroom trips decreased by 79 percent in patients on colostrum-based supplement compared to a 58 percent reduction in controls. Self-reported fatigue was reduced by 85 percent in patients on colostrum-based supplement by week 9 compared to 43 percent reduction among controls. Patients on colostrum-based supplement had 11 percent increase in mean body weight and body mass index by week 9 but no changes were observed in control subjects. Mean CD4+ count increased by 14 percent for patients on colostrum-based supplement in contrast to 12 percent decrease in controls. "This study shows that addition of colostrum-based supplement to standard therapy is effective in treatment of HIV-associated diarrhea."

In a study carried out at Braithwaite Memorial Specialist Hospital, Port Harcourt, Nigeria, 30 patients with HIV-associated diarrhea were included in the study. The patients were treated with colostrum for four weeks in an open-label non-randomized study after an observational period of one week. There was a dramatic decrease in bathroom trips, substantial decrease in self-estimated fatigue of 81 percent, increase in body-weight of 7.3 kg per patient and an increase in CD4+ count by 125 percent. Thus colostrum "may be an important alternative or additional treatment in HIV-associated diarrhea." [20, 21, 22, 23, 24, 25]

PROTEIN BERRY SMOOTHIE

This is one of my favorite smoothies. I fill it with everything organic and everything powerful. As you will note I like to use water along with the coconut cream concentrate. But you can substitute the coconut cream concentrate with hemp granules, sunflower seeds or some almonds. You can also use almond milk, hemp milk or milk of your choice. I have found that products sweetened with xylitol go with bitter foods and/or less sweet fruits. This is why berries work so well with this recipe.

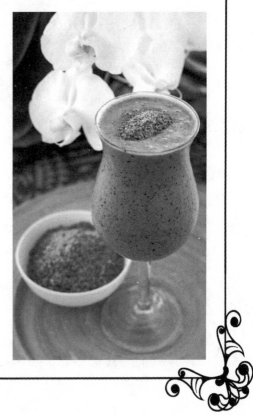

Fill the blender with water first and then all other ingredients, leaving the berries for last. I love to make this mixture thick and then pour it into a bowl, top with Barlean's Forti Flax and eat it with a spoon. I feel like I get an ice-cream fix, but better.

8 oz	water
1 T	Immune-Tree Colostrum6
1 T	coconut cream concentrate (or coconut oil)
1	scoop PhytoPro Organic Protein—Vanilla
1	scoop Barlean's Greens
1 C	frozen berries of choice, or other fruits
	pinch salt
	ice as desired

REPAIRING THE LEAKY GUT

For centuries, colostrum has been one of the world's most revered foods. But where it excels in its effects is on the gastrointestinal tissues. For anyone with gastrointestinal problems—especially leaky gut syndrome as well as anyone taking non-steroidal anti-inflammatory drugs or who drinks alcohol, which damage the gut lining—colostrum could be a lifesaver.

In fact, if you are taking a baby aspirin a day or using other non-steroidal anti-inflammatory drugs (NSAIDs) such as ibuprofen, this information is critical. And if you imbibe alcohol, once again, you will find that colostrum is a lifesaver.

DAMAGED GUT—SERIOUS, WIDESPREAD

"A major task of the intestine is to form a defensive barrier to prevent absorption of damaging substances from the external environment," says Daniel Hollander, MD, of Harbor-UCLA Research and Education Institute, and one of the nation's inflammatory bowel disease experts.[26]

This protective yet versatile in-and-out function of the intestinal mucosa is called permeability. Clinicians use inert, nonmetabolized sugars such as mannitol, rhamnose, or lactulose to measure the permeability barrier or the degree of leakiness of the intestinal mucosa.

Ample evidence indicates that permeability is increased in most patients with Crohn's disease and in 10-20% of their clinically healthy relatives.

Permeability is also increased in celiac disease and by trauma, burns and use of even some low-dose NSAIDs (aspirin users).

Leaky gut is linked to liver disease. Only 30% of alcoholics develop cirrhosis, suggesting that the development of alcohol-induced liver injury requires one or more additional factors, say researchers at the Department of Medicine (Division of Gastroenterology), Loyola University Medical School, Maywood, Illinois. Animal studies have shown that gut-derived endotoxin is one such factor. Because increased intestinal permeability has been shown to cause endotoxemia, they now believe increased gastrointestinal permeability (leaky gut) contributes to alcoholic liver disease. "Because only the alcoholics with chronic liver disease had increased intestinal permeability, we conclude that a 'leaky' gut may be a necessary cofactor for the development of chronic liver injury in heavy drinkers."[27]

LEAKY GUT INFLAMMATION

Inflammation causes damage to the gastrointestinal tissue, resulting in excess permeability and unusually large spaces between the cells of the mucosal lining, which allows bacteria, viruses, fungi and other potentially toxic materials to enter the bloodstream. The widened spaces can also allow undigested food particles to "leak" through the intestinal lining. This could pose a serious health risk since these particles may be considered "foreign" by the body and the immune system may try to destroy them.

Many of the pathogens that make us sick enter the body through the food we eat. This means that an individual with leaky gut syndrome is much more vulnerable to infection than someone with a healthy gastrointestinal tract.

The activation of immune cells within the huge surface area of the gut lining can cause a systemic inflammatory response—and overall bodily inflammation, we now are learning, is linked with heart disease, cancer, arthritis and diabetes. The passage of bacteria and toxins through leaky gut mucosa may amplify or perpetuate this systemic inflammation.[28]

First milk can be of value to anyone at risk for leaky gut. The immune factors in colostrum contain a number of antibodies that bind to invading microorganisms and hold them in check while they are destroyed by white blood cells.

The most important of these antibodies are of the IgA type. Not only do they attach themselves to an invading microorganism they are also able to *stick* to tissues, making it easier for white blood cells to search out and destroy the immobilized pathogen. The process of destroying invading microorganisms is aided by other substances present in colostrum. These include lactoferrin and transferrin, which capture the iron required by some bacteria to reproduce. Also, several enzymes in colostrum are capable of eating holes in the walls of various microorganisms.

The growth factors in colostrum are also of substantial benefit in leaky gut syndrome. It is documented that growth hormone and the insulinlike growth factor superfamily of proteins, both of which are found in abundance in first-milking colostrum, aid in the proliferation of new cells.

These and other factors in colostrum can actually repair the damaged mucosal tissues. Recent studies have documented how the use of bovine colostrum reduces excess permeability caused by the use of NSAIDS. The repair of the mucosal lining may also decrease the severity of some food allergies—especially associated with undigested food particles leaking into the bloodstream.

Irene Ballosh, Del Rio, Texas, wrote me, "For several years, I was plagued with digestive problems. It had gotten to the point where I practically lived on goat's milk, and I couldn't even touch vegetables—cooked or raw. I took digestive enzymes, which helped very little, and nothing seemed to help the severe pain, bloating and gas that would result when I ate. My doctor, who had received significant benefits from colostrum, suggested I take it. I was skeptical, but I agreed to take three capsules twice a day. Within a month, I noticed that my stomach didn't hurt anymore and that I felt better, so just to see how much better I really was, I made myself a salad with all the things that used to give me the most trouble. I included lettuce, bell peppers, raw onions and carrots. Any one of those would have caused terrible pain and suffering the month before, but I didn't experience any difficulty. Today, I can eat anything I want. The other thing colostrum has done for me is build up my immune system. This winter I never even got a sniffle. I have gradually increased the amount of colostrum I take—more than doubling the original dosage and my blood sugar has normalized in the past year. I have been able to eliminate the medication I used to take for diabetes. This is something I didn't realize colostrum could do, until recently. I consider first-milking colostrum to be a minor miracle in my life!"

Lawrence Lightfritz told me about his ulcerative colits. He suffered four years. "During the last year it had gotten so bad, with diarrhea and bleeding, that I literally had to go the bathroom 20 times a day—bleeding every time. I couldn't eat anything that was the least bit spicy or greasy without severe complications. Doctors had tried several different medications.

"None of them worked at all. I was so tired and run down that if I hadn't discovered colostrum, I don't know where I would be today. Within two weeks of taking six capsules per day I could tell a difference. The bleeding and diarrhea were noticeably less severe. Within a month, the bleeding had stopped and I had a nearly normal, firm stool. After two months, I have two normal bowel movements per day and I can eat anything I want again. I feel absolutely great! The other interesting thing is that I have tried three different brands of colostrum. Two of them did nothing. Only when I take the first-milking brand, do the symptoms subside and stay in check."

"I have had irritable bowel syndrome for six years, but when I started taking first-milking colostrum, it began to help right away," says Barbara Chittenden. "After only five days, my symptoms were gone. I still can't believe it. I have gone from being bloated most of the time, with cramping and diarrhea, to being completely free of digestive distress. I have also lost weight."

CAFÉ COLOSTRUM

1t - T   Mate, green tea, black tea or coffee
1 t   Immune-Tree Colostrum6
           Barlean's Organic Cococnut Oil
           XyloSweet, honey or maple syrup to taste

Brew your favorite hot beverage and pour into a blender. Add Immune-Tree Colostrum6 and coconut oil. Blend until frothy. Using Colostrum6 for a creamer is one of the anti-agers you can give for your body and your palate. The enhancement of the flavor and what it does for the health of your palate and the rest of you are profoundly different from any other cream I've ever used. It makes my tea and coffee so darn delicious I swoon with every sip.

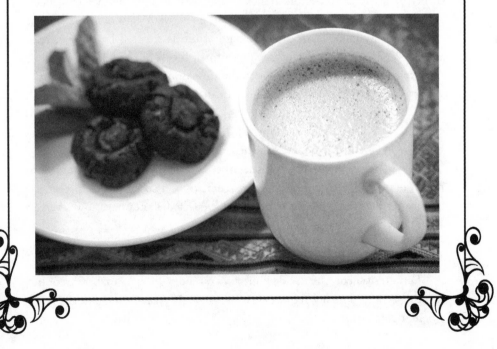

7

HEALTHY BLOOD SUGAR

The best-known and most common metabolic disorder is diabetes mellitus, a disease caused by defective carbohydrate metabolism and characterized by abnormally high levels of sugar in the blood and urine. It can eventually result in damage to the eyes, kidneys, heart and limbs.

There are two types of diabetes. Type I is called insulin-dependent diabetes mellitus (IDDM), previously known as juvenile-onset diabetes since it occurs primarily in children and young adults. It accounts for about 10 to 15 percent of all cases of diabetes and can progress very rapidly. Type II is called non-insulin-dependent diabetes mellitus (NIDDM), formerly known as adult-onset diabetes since it usually occurs in those over 40 years of age. This form of diabetes progresses slowly and individuals often have no outward signs of illness.

In healthy individuals, the hormone insulin is secreted by the pancreas. Insulin regulates the entry of glucose into each cell in the body. Glucose is then converted into glycogen (under the direction of IGF-1), providing the energy required for bodily functions. In diabetes, this process is impaired, either because of insufficient insulin in the body (Type I) or an inability to convert glucose to glycogen (Type II). In either case, sugar builds up in the blood and is eventually excreted in the urine.

It is unclear exactly what causes either type of diabetes, but it does seem to run in families and Type II diabetes seems to be associated with prolonged obesity. In addition, people with either type of diabetes have low levels of IGF-1 in their circulation.

The American Diabetes Association has estimated that 1 in every 14 people in the United States either have, or will have, diabetes during their lifetime.

Diabetes is generally divided into two categories. Type I diabetes requires insulin. Type II does not require insulin although it can develop to the point where it is required.

Type I diabetes is often referred to as juvenile onset diabetes and can progress rapidly. Frequently, it develops as an autoimmune disease where antibodies attack the insulin-producing cells of the pancreas. One early treatment for this form of diabetes is the use of immunosuppressive drugs, which may cause other complications. As a viable alternative, colostrum contains a substance known as proline-rich polypeptide, shown to balance the overactive immune response associated with autoimmune diseases (see Chapter 5). Rather than suppressing the immune system with drugs, colostrum can stimulate suppressor and helper immune cells from the thymus that tamp down overactive immune responses to reduce the attack on pancreatic cells.

Diabetes requires careful dietary and exercise programs. Even though Type II is a milder form, it is not without secondary complications, including heart and kidney disease, atherosclerosis, vision and circulatory problems. Those with diabetes, regardless of the type, are five times more likely to develop cardiovascular disease than those without. Often diabetes is diagnosed for the first time following a heart attack.

A 1990 publication in *Diabetes* suggested colostrum supplementation for diabetes based on the fact that IGF-1 can stimulate glucose utilization. Researchers found that IGF-1 levels were lower in diabetic patients than in healthy individuals. After administering IGF-1 to patients, doctors noticed a two-fold increase in glucose transport to the muscles, potentially treating hyperglycemia and the dependence on insulin.

A study from *Clinical and Molecular Medicine*, Sapienza University of Rome, shows that the administration of colostrum benefits the subjects with type 2 diabetes mellitus as it gradually regulates appetite and improves utilization of nutrients, especially glucose, which leads to a significant decrease in body fat. Their study aimed at verifying a possible reduction in the use of insulin in 27 subjects with type 2 diabetes who were treated with colostrum in the form of gastro-resistant tablets of 300 mg.

In subjects with type 2 diabetes treated with insulin, the administration of colostrum "obtained a significant reduction of insulin dosage and normalization of blood glucose levels." The effects of colostrum are presumably linked to increased levels of IGF-1 "that improves the utilization of glucose, stimulates glycogen and protein synthesis."

Daily supplementation with high quality first milking bovine colostrum can help restore a diabetic's diminished levels of IGF-1, increasing the utilization of available glucose. This becomes extremely important for the Type I diabetic who receives routine injections of insulin. The IGF-1 in colostrum can assure effective and controlled utilization of available glucose once the individual's insulin levels are restored. In the Type II diabetic, where sufficient insulin is available, experiments have shown that restoring IGF-1 levels in the blood resulted in reduced glucose levels in the blood and urine, indicating an improvement in glucose utilization by the body.

A note of caution: Colostrum is not a panacea and the restoration of IGF-1 levels alone will not "cure" diabetes. Colostrum supplementation must be coupled with a controlled dietary program and routine exercise. Although some individuals have been able to reduce or eliminate the use of insulin by taking colostrum, any modification in medication should be strictly supervised by a qualified health professional.

The Graham family discovered colostrum while searching for something to help Yvonne's 8-year-old niece who had been recently diagnosed with juvenile diabetes. They were disturbed by the sudden diagnosis and concerned with the amount of insulin being given a young child with no hope for anything else... Everything Yvonne read about colostrum made so much sense that she contacted her sister and shared her discovery. Yvonne found a "first-milking" colostrum with very high levels of immune and growth factors and her niece started taking it along with several other suporting supplements. Yvonne says, "At first we got really scared because her blood sugar went up, but we had been told blood sugar levels might fluctuate while the body was finding a new balance, so we kept giving her the colostrum. Within a short period of time there was marked improvement and insulin levels were reduced. After three months there were no insulin requirements at all—none!"

"For five to six years I have struggled with hypoglycemia," says Charles Ruiz. "Nearly every day, several hours after lunch, I would feel its effects. I would get woozy and often have to sit down until it passed. Not anymore. I have been taking colostrum for a little over five months and the afternoon hypoglycemia attacks have ceased completely. My blood sugar levels are in the normal range again. Also, for the first time in my life, I didn't get sick at all during the winter and my allergies have been noticeably milder this summer."

Cassie York, age 80, says, "I have been on insulin for at least 30 years. In the last several years my need for insulin had increased and I was receiving two injections per day. The circulation in my leg had become so poor that I needed a cane to get around. My leg was turning black and crusty and doctors were beginning to discuss amputation at the knee. In March, I began taking colostrum. Surprisingly, within one month, my morning sugar was no longer elevated and week by week, as I had my blood sugar tested, my need for insulin became less and less. Now, I no longer require insulin injections at all. I take one pill a day and that seems to be enough. Even better than that is the fact that the color has begun to return in my leg and doctors are no longer talking about amputation. I don't have headaches anymore. I have lost weight and the skin under my chin has tightened up."

"I have diabetes, fibromyalgia, osteoporosis and osteoarthritis, any one of which can be debilitating," Pat Bailye says. "I was so depressed and so sick for almost two years that I didn't really care anymore. When I began taking colostrum, I worked up to six capsules per day. The first thing I noticed was that my appetite changed. (With diabetes, you can eat a big meal and still feel hungry.) I noticed that after several weeks on the colostrum I didn't feel hungry any more. I noticed that my energy was increasing and that I wasn't as depressed. Then I noticed that my blood sugar levels were changing. With careful monitoring (two to four times a day), I have been able to lower my insulin from 96 units per day to 10 units per day during the last nine months. I used to take lots of pain medication—now I take none; a good warm bath is all I need to help with occasional pain from overwork. I am working again and supporting myself after two years of not being able to. All this didn't happen at once, so I would encourage people to have patience."

HOW TO USE

"As a naturopathic physician, I was using colostrum 20 years ago," says Thomas Stone, ND. "Back then, I could get it from organic farmers in the Midwest. Today, I recommend first-milking colostrum in capsules and lozenges. For diabetic patients, within months, everyone either greatly reduces levels of insulin or they have eliminated the need altogether. That's quite a track record, but it's true." Of course, they are also drinking plenty of good water, exercising and eating an enhanced diet of "live whole foods," but it is the colostrum that makes the program work, he adds.

"Given time, colostrum can in some cases eliminate the need for insulin. It balances the pancreas just like it does the thymus so that blood sugar levels are able to normalize." However, for all prospective users, particularly insulin-dependent patients, it is very important to consult a health care practitioner before taking colostrum or making changes in medication.

ALMOND/FLAX CELERY BUTTER

Place Colostrum6 in a bowl and add Barlean's Flax Oil, pressing the mixture together with a spoon to blend. This dissolves any potential lumps. When smooth, add in the almond butter and blend. Fill celery sticks with this yummy butter and enjoy! You can also serve with carrots and an assorted vegetable tray.

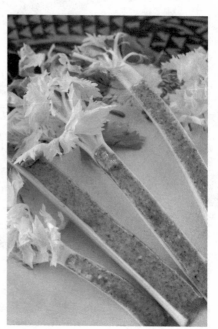

1 T   Immune-Tree Colostrum6

2-3 T   almond butter

1 T   Barlean's Flax Oil

         Celery sticks or assorted veggies

NIGHTTIME WEIGHT LOSS FACTOR

You can lose weight and build muscles while...sleeping. Leptin regulates the brain's receptors for sugar and fat storage; it tells the brain how much the body has of each and how much it needs. But it gets suppressed with obesity and sometimes it takes the addition of extra leptin to resignal the brain that the body has enough fat stores and sugar. People who've used colostrum with leptin say it takes the edge off of their nighttime hunger pangs. You won't need to buy special foods. You will just spend less money on food because you won't be as hungry and instead enjoy your portions more with less overeating or midnight snacking. Your body ends up not craving sugar or salt and the pounds melt off. Most people drink their leptin shakes in the morning or have one at night.

OBESITY CLINICS TEST LEPTIN

A randomized, controlled trial performed at six different obesity clinics looked at the effects of leptin on 73 obese men and women. Researchers reported in *The Journal of the American Medical Association* that daily use of leptin led to a mean weight loss of 15 pounds in a 24-week treatment period. More than 95% of the lost weight was from body fat.

There was considerable variation in the amount of weight that individual subjects lost during the treatment. Subjects who took the highest daily doses of leptin also lost the most weight.

Many studies show that colostrum's natural enveloping of the leptin molecule and other potentially fragile peptides and proteins actually shepherds the compounds through the gastrointestinal tract and into the bloodstream where it does the most good.

All this should really come as no surprise when you know that the word leptin comes from the Greek word leptos, meaning "thin."

This protein hormone, discovered in 1994, regulates body weight and metabolism. It is expressed predominantly by adipocytes, the fancy word for fat cells, and acts like a signal to the brain on the status of fat stores elsewhere in the body; the hypothalamus, it turns out, has leptin receptors where they attach to regulate food intake and body weight.

Leptin appears to lead to a dramatic reduction in food intake and to as much as a 50% reduction in body weight within months. Along with decreased food consumption, there is an increase in the body's energy expenditure, which in turn leads to a loss of fat tissue mass and an increase in lean muscle.

Researchers discovered in 2000 that when leptin works in conjunction with IGF-1 and other cofactors found in colostrum; it can also shrink fat cells to normal size. (IGF-1 directs the body's metabolic process, burning fat, balancing blood sugar and building lean muscle.)

Research on the body's obesity (*ob*) gene and leptin thus far have assumed that the protein acts by causing a hormonal response in the brain, leading one to feel satiated. Purdue University Professor Ki-Han Kim, however, has discovered these findings are only partly correct. He says the body's sense of sweetness declines with leptin deficit, and production in fat cells slows. Leptin, known as the fat-burning hormone, is intimately tied into the body's ability to resist sweet treats, by turning on and off particular genetic characteristics that allow the tongue to taste sugar. The tongue was found to be one of the peripheral targets for leptin.

The finding gives scientists the first indication that leptin suppresses biochemical reactions in fat cells without the participation of the brain.

When researchers injected laboratory mice with leptin, previously obese mice ones as thin as rodent track stars. "It's true that the animal isn't eating as much when it is given leptin," Kim says. "But that doesn't mean that the brain is initiating this. Whenever we eat, we alter the hormonal status of the body. The body has to tell its various parts to do something with this food that has been ingested. When leptin inhibits fat synthesis, it causes the body to have extra food in its system, which triggers the hormonal system to send a message to the brain saying that the body is satiated and to stop eating. So leptin's interaction in the brain isn't the whole story. Leptin also appears to act via pathways that are independent of the brain. My thinking is that it works by inhibiting the synthesis of fat in fat cells and increasing the burning of fat in muscle cells. It works at an enzymatic, cellular level."

Kim found that the *ob* gene causes the muscle cells to produce leptin and suppresses another gene that produces an enzyme known as acetyl-CoA carboxylase, or ACC, essential for fat production.

To capture the power of leptin, colostrum is one of nature's richest sources, note researchers from the University of Milan reporting in *Hormone and Metabolic Research.* They studied leptin content in bovine colostrum and concluded that, "leptin is present in large quantities in colostrum..."[29]

Colostrum also contains IGF-1, which is required to metabolize fat for energy, thus supporting the effect of leptin's impact on caloric control. The effect of colostrum is to increase lean muscle mass and decrease body fat simultaneously. The benefit is cumulative since increased muscle mass results in more calorie burning and conversion of fat to energy. Colostrum works while you dream. To experience truly great results, an inch loss program needs to work with your body 24 hours a day, 7 days a week, even while you sleep.

HOW TO USE WITH ADDITIONAL WEIGHT-LOSS NUTRIENTS

Leptin-enriched colostrum formulas also can contain citrus extract, raspberry ketones and green tea, a combination with some scientific evidence for appetite inhibition and weight loss.[30]

Raspberry ketones, an aromatic component, cause fat breakdown. In one experiment, to test the effect on obesity, mice were fed a high-fat diet plus raspberry ketones for about 10 weeks. Researchers observed that, compared to controls, raspberry ketones decreased the amount of fat in the liver and visceral adipose (abdominal fat) tissues of mice. It also significantly increased norepinephrine-induced lipolysis (the decomposition of fat) in cells. Researchers also tested fat cells with raspberry ketones and found that they showed greater evidence of breakdown when compared to controls. Be forewarned, however. In order to consume enough of the ketones in raspberries, requires a nutritional supplement—or else consumption of about 90 pounds of the fruit daily.

The Journal of Medicine notes that *Citrus aurantium* is a weight-loss herb, working as a beta agonist. The researchers reported increased metabolic rates and significant weight loss when ingesting *Citrus aurantium* products. At present, *Citrus aurantium* may be the best thermogenic substitute for ephedra. However, more studies are needed to establish this.[31]

In another randomized, placebo-controlled, double-blind study, 70 obese but otherwise healthy subjects were assigned to receive citrus extracts, raspberry ketones and green tea or a placebo and underwent eight weeks of daily supplementation, a calorie restricted diet and exercise training. Of the 45 subjects who completed the study, significant positive differences were observed in: body weight, fat mass, lean mass, waist girth, hip girth and energy levels as well as serum leptin.

Usually the loss of weight is an added surprise for those who take colostrum. Both GH and IGF-I play a significant role in the body's ability to burn fat and build lean muscle.

A report from the University Clinic of Internal Medicine in Denmark concluded that GH prevents the body from burning glucose for energy and, instead, increases fat oxidation. GH also acts as a catalyst in the production of IGF-I, which is involved in nutrient uptake and the growth of muscle cells. Tests conducted in Sweden on elderly adults, who had low amounts of lean muscle mass and had lost strength and exercise capacity, noted distinct improvement when supplemented with GH. It was also observed that even though muscle mass increased, overall weight did *not*. This indicates that fat was burned as muscle was gained. The interactive influence of both GH and IGF-I has a major influence on metabolism. Together, GH and IGF-I restore many important metabolic processes in the aging body. This often results in a decrease in body fat and a shift from fat to lean muscle tissue.

"[When I started taking colostrum,] I didn't realize it would help me lose weight but I have been able to lose 20 pounds during the last 3 months without changing my diet," says Pete D. "I used to play football in college but ever since I quit, I have put on a little more weight each year. Three months ago I weighed 250 pounds. Now I am down to 230—without even trying."

Janet D. writes she "took about 11,000 milligrams of first-milking colostrum per day for several months before reducing to a lesser amount, which I am committed to take regularly. I have also had some marvelous success with slimming down. I have lost inches without altering my diet."

ORANGE LIME VANILLA DREAM

Combine all ingredients and blend until creamy and frothy. These ingredients deliver a creamy texture with fresh bold flavor with hemp seeds for essential fatty acids, fresh juice for vitamin C and other nutrients, lecithin and colostrum for cell repair and renewal and immunity, protein for strength and stamina and vanilla-flavored protein powder. YUM!

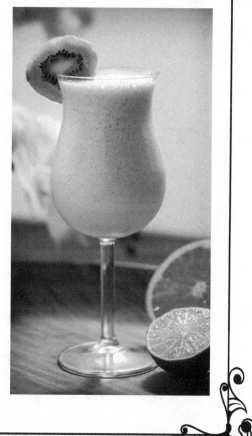

1	scoop MHP Probolic-SR Vanilla
1/3 C	hemp seeds
2 T	coconut cream concentrate
½ C	orange juice
1/3 C	lime juice or the juice of one lime
1 T	soy lecithin granules
1 T	Immune-Tree Colostrum6
1 C	water (approximately)
	ice

DENTAL HEALTH

Researchers from the Institute of Dentistry and Turku Immunology Center, at the University of Turku, Finland, have studied the effect of colostrum on dental and oral health.[32]

Colostrum from cows immunized with the cavity-causing bacterium *Mutans streptococci* was used as a mouth rinse in a short-term human study. Since it was a colostrum from cows purposefully exposed to the bacterium, it was rich in *Mutans streptococci*-specific antibodies. The relative number of *Mutans streptococci* in the oral cavity "significantly decreased" with this special colostrum, the researchers found. "Thus," they note, short term rinsing indicates "favourable effects" of bovine immune colostrum on human dental plaque.

"Bovine antibodies may also provide protection against dental caries," notes Professor Hannu Korhonen of the Agricultural Research Center, Jokioinen, Finland. Immune milk concentrate "has significant antimetabolic potential against *S. mutans*," the main cause of caries and "actively inhibits *in vitro* the adherence of these bacteria to hydroxyapatite and supports the natural antimicrobial systems present in the saliva."

So far, only a few clinical human trials have been reported on the use of anti-cavity colostrum antibodies derived from colostrum of hyperimmunized cows. "The results obtained encourage continuation of such studies and development of innovative commercial products, which contain active antibodies," says Dr. Korhonen.

STICKS TO GUMS

For dental health, prefer powdered colostrum. The tendency of first-milking colostrum to stick to the gums like a paste and slowly dissolve is beneficial. You see, there's more to colostrum than simply being a rich source of anti-bacterial antibodies. Its growth factors and immune components work together to influence oral health.

I base this on research, which shows that colostrum has rejuvenating effects on the gastrointestinal membrane. In fact, so remarkable is its ability to restore the integrity of the gastrointestinal lining that colostrum is now being recommended by doctors to their patients who are taking typical painkillers, such as aspirin and ibuprofen (see Chapter 6). I believe colostrum has similar beneficial effects on the gums. The many growth factors in colostrum strengthen the lining of the gums, rejuvenating their vitality.

The human mouth is one of the main routes of entry of foreign microorganisms into the body and, therefore, orally transmitted diseases are widespread and common in human populations. Colostrum appears to also enhance saliva-mediated protection against dental diseases as well as other orally transmitted infections.

Responsible also for gum disease, the bacterium *Porphyomonas gingivitis* is now also known for its damaging effects on the linings of the arteries. According to the work of Dr. Raul Garcia of the Boston VA Outpatient Clinic and part of the VA Normative Aging Study, over a 25-year period some 1,100 men were studied. They were healthy at the start, but the men with the worst gums had twice the heart-attack rate of their peers with healthy gums and odorless breath. Their stroke rate was three times as high. The bacterium has also been found at the scene of the crime: in diseased carotid arteries.

So you see by taking care of your dental health with colostrum, you're also taking care of many other aspects of your health.

LEMON YOGURT CAKE

(Gluten Free & Sugar Free)

Cake Batter:

1 C	gluten free flour (or flour of choice)
½ t	baking powder
1 C	XyloSweet
1 C	whole milk plain yogurt
2	eggs
2	lemons (zest only) juice lemons for frosting/drizzle Pinch salt

Drizzle:

1 C	lemon juice
½ C	XyloSweet
¼ C	Immune-Tree Colostrum6
1 T	cornstarch
1 T	water

Mix lemon juice, XyloSweet and Colostrum6 in a blender. When it is thoroughly blended, add water and corn starch. Move to sauce pan and bring to a boil. The drizzle will thicken quickly. Add water as needed. Let the mixture cool and drizzle over cake when it has cooled slightly. Note: I added a tiny sprinkle of turmeric to the drizzle to bring up the color. As you can see it became a little bright. Coloring is optional.

Mix all the dry ingredients together (flour, baking soda and XyloSweet) and lemon zest. Beat eggs and yogurt together until smooth and add to dry mixture. Blend thoroughly. Pour batter into cake pan of choice and bake at 350 degrees for 70 minutes. Check color after 40 to 50 minutes and cover the cake with foil if it is getting too brown. Remove the cake from the oven and let cool before transferring to a plate or frosting.

10

FIRST MILK AS ALZHEIMER'S VACCINE

5.4m	16m	130bln	41.8%
Americans with Alzheimer's disease	people projected to have disease by 2050	in Medicare and Medicaid spending for Alzheimer's disease in 2011	of residents with Alzheimer's / dementias in assisted living and other residential care

No one expects a cure for Alzheimer's disease anytime soon. Most of the drugs currently on the market for AD are inhibitors of the enzyme that breaks down the brain transmitter acetylcholine after it has been produced by nerve cells. But what if the nerve cells are dying and there is not enough acetylcholine? In the October 2013 issue of *Science Translational Medicine*, scientists at the University of Leicester said their genetic influencing compound switched off defective processes that lead to death of brain cells. "We're still a long way from a usable drug for humans—this compound had serious side effects," Giovanna Mallucci, one of the study researchers, said. "But the fact that we have established that this pathway can be manipulated to protect against brain cell loss, first with genetic tools and now with a compound, means that developing drug treatments targeting this pathway for... neurodegenerative diseases is now a real possibility."

Colostrum is the source of a compound research shows can halt the progression of Alzheimer's disease (AD) and is regenerative to the human body.

Actual colostrum, which isn't synthetic, doesn't work by inhibiting acetylcholine destruction but by renewing and restoring brain cells. The first milk contains proline-rich polypeptide or PRP; studied clinically in Europe, it "holds therapeutic interest" for Alzheimer's prevention, say Drs. M Janusz and A Zablocka in the November 2013 issue of *Cellular Molecular Biology*.[33] They say this mixture of peptides derived from colostrum could help slow the progression of Alzheimer's disease by reducing the build-up of beta amyloid, a toxic protein that accumulates in the brains of sufferers.

In July 2009 the *Journal of Nutritional Health and Aging* noted neuronal cells pretreated with PRPs avoid the accumulation of beta-amyloid. A review article in the October 1, 2007 issue of *Progress in Neuro-Psychopharmacology and Biological Psychiatry* by A. Gladkevich of the Department of Psychiatry, University Groningen, the Netherlands, concluded: "Both experimental and clinical evidence support a beneficial effect of proline-rich polypeptides in a number of neurodegenerative diseases, including Alzheimer disease."

These studies offer explanations for the early promising results at The Psychiatric Unit, University Medical School, Wroclaw, Poland. There 46 AD patients were divided into 3 groups and randomly assigned to receive orally either colostrum tablets, selenium or placebo. Eight of the 15 AD patients treated with the colostrum "improved and in the 7 others the disease had stabilized. In contrast, none of the 31 patients from the selenium or placebo groups with similar mild or moderate AD improved."[34]

Technically speaking, proline-rich polypeptides or PRPs, isolated from first-milking colostrum, are tiny amino acid sequences consisting of ten chains or less made up of high amounts of proline. Though tiny, they are critical to healthy immune function and activate the thymus gland to produce mature T cells including T helper and suppressor cells that balance out inflammatory cascades. Their restorative powers were later found to extend to neurons.

Daily diet is as easy as adding a super food to your anti-aging program. Use the recipes in this book or eat by the spoonful. A lot of people find first-milking colostrum powder additive--and there's nothing wrong with this addiction. Therapeutically, working with yours or your loved one's doctor. When using as a dietary supplement, take or administer three 500 mg capsules of first-milking colostrum 3x times daily with meals.

CAFÉ CACAO

Immune-Tree's Colostrum6 has changed my tea and coffee routine. Finally, here is powerful substitution for cream. In this café cacao drink, it is the Colostrum6 that provides the thick texture and foam, the coconut oil that gives it a fat and richness for your brain and skin, and a hint of cacao to further the high powered experience.

1 C	freshly brewed organic coffee
1 T	Immune-Tree Colostrum6
1 T	Barlean's Coconut Oil
1 t	cacao powder
	pinch cardamom
	and cinnamon

Blend all of the ingredients together until foamy. Enjoy! Bet you can't drink just one!

11

HEART HEALTH

The heart is a hollow muscular organ that receives blood from the veins and then propels it out through the arteries. The blood carries oxygen, nutrients and immune factors to all parts of the body. All of the cells and organs in our body need oxygen and nutrients to function properly. If blood flow is disrupted, body cells can die and organs can be damaged, sometimes with deadly results.

One major form of heart disease is atherosclerosis, a condition where deposits called plaque, composed of cholesterol and fatty acids (triglycerides), build up on the inner wall of the coronary arteries. As plaque builds up, the arteries narrow, restricting blood flow to the heart. Symptoms of restricted blood flow can include shortness of breath, particularly during exercise and a tightening pain in the chest called *angina pectoris*. The plaque may become large enough to cause an occlusion, completely obstructing the coronary artery and depriving a portion of the heart of oxygen. Alternatively, some of the plaque may break off and lodge itself at another site, also causing a blockage. This is called a thrombosis. Both of these events are major causes of heart attacks and are often fatal.

Individuals with high serum cholesterol are most at risk for atherosclerosis and often have to monitor their dietary intake of cholesterol. Bovine colostrum does not contain cholesterol and can be used safely by individuals with high serum cholesterol and high triglycerides. In fact, there are biologically active substances present in colostrums that could be very beneficial to individuals at risk for atherosclerotic plaque formation. For instance, bovine colostrum contains leptin and insulin, which work together to promote healthy fat metabolism, potentially reducing serum cholesterol levels.

Two other forms of heart disease usually found in older individuals include pulmonary heart disease and congestive heart failure. Pulmonary heart disease is usually the result of a lung ailment, such as emphysema, or a disease affecting blood circulation to the lungs such as atherosclerosis of the pulmonary artery. In persons afflicted with congestive heart failure, the ventricles pump blood less efficiently than normal and the muscular walls of the ventricles enlarge in an effort to send more blood into the circulation. This gives rise to large, floppy hearts in such individuals.

The growth hormone and IGF-1 in bovine colostrum are weapons for combating cardiovascular disease. Receptors for both growth hormone and IGF-1 are found on all heart muscle cells, and scientific evidence indicates that growth hormone may act directly on the heart. These two growth factors work together to stimulate healthy heart muscle growth. In addition, IGF-1 and growth hormone can actually induce repair of damaged heart tissue. Administration of growth hormone to patients with congestive heart failure can result in a marked improvement in heart function and clinical status.

At the time he was diagnosed with congestive heart failure, Arlan Reynolds had already had other heart problems but he had somehow been able to maintain his work and his outside interests.

However, congestive heart failure meant limiting physical exertion for the rest of his life. Arlan notes, "I was told that I had an enlarged heart—that there was a certain percentage of it that was actually 'dead.' I was given very little hope of ever having a normal life again." When he discovered colostrum and began taking it, Arlan had no expectation for what might happen. He faithfully took eight to ten capsules per day and he continued with his regular nutritional program. As time went on, he noticed an increase in energy and stamina but he had no idea what was really happening until 18 months later when he went in for his annual physical exam. "My doctor took X-rays of my heart along with other routine tests," says Arlan. "He compared the X-rays with the ones which had originally been taken. Then he sent me to a special facility to have his findings substantiated. After numerous other tests, including more X-rays, an EKG and an echo-cardiogram, the doctor told me that he didn't understand what had taken place, but that all the tests indicated my heart had returned to normal size. My doctor said that in all his years of practice, he had never seen an enlarged heart return to normal size." Arlan's next question to the doctor was, "Are you telling me that I can play racquetball again?" The doctor's reply was simply, "I would highly recommend it."

HOW TO USE

First-milking colostrum can be enjoyed as a smoothie ingredient with two servings daily recommended. When using as a dietary supplement, take three 500 mg capsules of first-milking colostrum 3x times daily with meals.

HI PROTEIN BLUE BERRY PANCAKES

Cake Batter:

½ C	oats
2	eggs
2 T	coconut milk
½	scoop MHP Protein Powder Vanilla Flavored
1 T	Immune-Tree Colostrum 6
2 C	Frozen or fresh blue berries
1 T	Barlean's Coconut Oil
	pinch of salt

Drizzle:

1 T	Barlean's Highest Lignan Flax Oil or Coconut Oil (or mix them)
1 t +	XyloSweet

The best way to make up the batter is to add the oats to the blender first, blending lightly into a powder. Then add the eggs, coconut milk, salt and blend again. Add in the protein powder and Immune-Tree Colostrum6 and give the blender a few more whirls. Your batter is now ready. Add a little water if more liquid is needed. Warm a skillet and add coconut oil. Pour batter into the hot skillet and grill up your cakes. When the last cake is out, toss the blueberries into the hot skillet and turn the heat off. It is OK if the blueberries are frozen. They will defrost quickly and begin to juice up a bit. Sprinkle in the XyloSweet. Remove the berries from the skillet and place on the top of the cakes. Pour the flax and/or coconut oil over the top. Both together are delicious.

12

SPORTS PERFORMANCE

Olympic silver medalist Winthrop Graham began using first-milking colostrum after a knee injury in the 1996 Olympics. "It was a rather serious injury and doctors wanted to perform surgery, but I opted for a rehabilitation program," says Graham. Two years passed. But he was still having trouble recovering after running the hurdles. His knee would become stiff and prevent him from training consistently. "However, within two months after I began taking 12 colostrum a day, I could run the hurdles with no stiffness at all," he says. "That was something and I became a believer."

For Jeff Spreng, first-milking colostrum helped him to realize his body building dreams. "I always wanted to be a body builder, so I tried everything to gain weight and build muscle but nothing had any significant effect until I found colostrum," Spreng says. He began taking a half-teaspoon twice a day. "Right away I noticed how good I felt." He increased his workouts to six hours per day. Thanks to his enhanced recovery, he was able to train seven days a week, losing twenty-five pounds, adding lean muscle and, all in all, becoming one "ripped" dude.

"People stop me on the street and say, 'I don't mean to embarrass you but you have the most incredible body.' No one ever said that kind of thing to me before," he says. "Now it happens all the time. My friends who knew me can't believe I've lost weight because they can see I'm bigger. It's so excellent!"

These days, Jeff uses two to three heaping teaspoons of colostrum powder, four times per day and is devoted fulltime to body building.

"I am a tree surgeon and I do a lot of weight training to stay fit," notes David K. "I have tried a number of things, including a homeopathic form of human growth hormone, but I have never been able to really gain weight. My weight stayed relatively constant for 30 years, between 190 and 200 pounds until I started taking colostrum. After three months, I weighed 220 with no increase in body fat."

A growing body of evidence suggests that colostrum is food for weight training, running, power sports and anyone interested in getting in shape, maintaining exercise intensity, regular tough training and muscle gain.

COLOSTRUM FOR TISSUE REPAIR AND RECOVERY

Each time we exercise strenuously, we cause tiny tears in muscle tissue. The growth factors in colostrum help to quickly repair this damage, strengthening muscles. The regenerative effects of colostrum extend to nearly all structural cells of the body; in fact, IGF-1 is the best known compound for synthesis and repair of cartilage. Other compounds known as transforming growth factors A and B are known for their ability to enhance healing and for taking part in the synthesis and repair of both RNA and DNA.

Several years ago, the Finnish Olympic ski team, participated in a study involving colostrum.[35] Members of the team who took colostrum showed reduced muscle-cell damage on the fourth day following seven days of acute exercise. They also reported being less fatigued.

Colostrum works for athletic injuries, from those that occur on a day to day basis within the muscle to those of a more serious nature. Most athletes report quicker recovery without the same level of fatigue.

For athletes interested in enhanced physical performance, the scientific evidence supporting use of colostrum is noteworthy. Its high content of bioactive growth factors is generating interest among sports doctors. Growth factors are made up of short protein chains called polypeptides that play key regulatory roles in cell growth, replication, and differentiation. Growth factors support complex feedback loops between the immune, nervous and hormonal systems that maintain healthy homeostasis under normal circumstances.

"Aging of the body is dramatically affected by replacing both growth hormone and the IGF-1 Super Family and the effects have been documented the world over," says Dr Eng Huu, an osteopathic physician and assistant professor at the Lake Erie College of Osteopathic Medicine in Bradenton, Florida. "These small hormone-like substances are part of a superfamily of 87 additional IGF-binding proteins that influence many aspects of how all cells develop, function and maintain their youthfulness. The superfamily represents substances that not only direct processes within cells but also keep them under control. These play a role in our body's ability to reduce damage, repair and rebuild cells—conditions greatly necessary to maintain youthful vitality and health."

Human growth hormone is responsible for many effects on growth, physical development, immunity and metabolism. Produced and secreted by the pituitary gland, GH is released in pulses in response from signals from the hypothalamus during sleep. It exerts anabolic effects throughout the body favoring tissue, bone and muscle.

GH works in tandem with IGF-I, a peptide that declines with age. Over time these decreased levels have significant negative effects on fat deposition, immunity and energy. Both GH and its mediator IGF-I may actually treat the blueprint of aging, keeping the cells in as healthy a state as possible. The cells' ability to function depends on the genetic codes for all the proteins, hormones, and enzymes that make the cell run.

Both GH and IGF-I feed DNA. GH initiates transport of amino acids and nucleic acids into cells but IGF-I finishes the work and facilitates the transport of nucleic acids into the actual nucleus of the cell where the DNA resides, giving it the raw materials needed to repair damage and initiate healthy division.

One way to boost GH and IGF-1 is with first milk. In the *Journal of Applied Physiology* the purpose of this study was to examine the effects of bovine colostrum supplementation on serum IGF-I concentrations during a strength and speed training period. Nine male sprinters and jumpers underwent three randomized experimental training treatments of 8 days separated by 13 days.[36] Post-training increases were noticed for serum IGF-I compared with the placebo (normal milk whey). "It appears that a bovine colostrum supplement...may increase serum IGF-I concentration in athletes during strength and speed training."

"The future of nutritional science lies not in merely supporting one body system as if it functioned independently of the others but in a product that supports the major body systems simultaneously," says Dr. Eng Huu, an osteopathic physician and assistant professor at the Lake Erie College of Osteopathic Medicine in Bradenton, Florida, who labels colostrum "a unique discovery which is experiencing overwhelming success in helping to balance, strengthen, and support these systems."

BUILDS LEAN MUSCLE

One of the difficulties with achieving muscular development is preventing muscle breakdown. The exercise is required to build muscle can also be the thing that causes muscle breakdown. A true first-milking colostrum addresses both ends of this dilemma. It contains a whole complex of compounds to build lean muscle mass and burn fat rather than muscle. The same growth factors which work to build lean muscle also play a pivotal role in preventing muscle breakdown during exercise. During heavy workouts and in times of hunger, the body tends to burn protein instead of fat. Since IGF-I governs the synthesis of protein from amino acids, having an abundance of this factor in the system means that muscle need not be burned for fuel during heavy workouts. Rather, more fat is utilized.

AIDS STAMINA

Athletes require strength and stamina to compete. Anything that will enhance endurance and maximize fuel is certainly an asset. The growth factors contained in colostrum shift fuel utilization from carbohydrate to fat, actually preventing the body from burning glucose for energy.

Colostrum works to heal athletic injuries, including those that occur on a day-to-day basis among intensely training athletes, to those of a more serious nature. Most athletes report quicker recovery without the usual fatigue.

SUPPORTS IMMUNE SYSTEM

Athletes such as marathoners as well as bodybuilders are prone to infections and other illnesses since intense athletic endeavors actually depress the immune system immediately following a period of activity. Factors contained in colostrum can make a remarkable difference in an athletes' immune response. Both growth factors and immune factors continually work to strengthen the immune system so that vulnerability after exercise is less of an issue. Athletes who take colostrum experience shorter recovery times, indicating less "down time" for the immune system.

Even though growth factors are usually discussed separately from the immune factors in colostrum, they have interactive roles. Growth hormone is considered an immuno-stimulant because it helps the body produce antibodies, T-cells and other white blood cells. Together with IGF-1, GH has been used quite successfully to fight off infection. Both growth factors and immune factors in colostrum support an athlete's immune system, helping to compensate for the stress from heavy workouts.

Roger J. tells us, "I have had chronic fatigue for seven years. Besides the lack of energy. . . I also gradually lost the strength and stamina to exercise the way I had always done. Now, with colostrum I am running 2 ¼-4 miles, five days a week and also aggressively working out five days a week—without inflamation or other symptoms."

AIDS NUTRIENT UPTAKE

Colostrum mends the lining of the digestive tract where nutrient absorption takes place. Not only does this enhance nutrient uptake, it also prevents invading organisms from attaching to the intestinal lining and causing infection. This also explains the boost in energy that many people feel when they take colostrum. Especially in the longer distances, leaky gut becomes a problem. So colostrum becomes an endurance edge.

SPORTS PERFORMANCE

Let's look at some of the research into the link between supplementing with colostrum and physical fitness.

Better Performance & Lower Serum Creatine Kinase At the Center for Research in Education and Sports Science, at the University of South Australia, a double-blind, placebo controlled study was carried out to determine the effect of supplementation with a commercial bovine colostrum product on plasma IGF-I concentrations and endurance running performance.[36] In the study, 39 males, aged 18-35 years, completed an eight-week running program while consuming 60 grams per day of the colostrum or whey protein. All subjects followed dietary guidelines provided by the researchers and kept food diaries throughout the study period for subsequent dietary analysis. Although no differences in plasma IGF-1 concentrations were found between the groups at the start or end of the study, the colostrum group continued to improve its performance capacity after four weeks, while the performance of the placebo group reached a plateau. By the eighth week, the colostrum group was running further and doing more work than the placebo group. Also of note, athletes receiving colostrum displayed a strong trend over eight weeks to reduce the increase in serum creatine kinase concentrations per unit of work done, while there was no such trend in the whey group. This is cutting-edge information. Creatine kinase is an enzyme that, during muscular activity, causes the breakdown of phosphocreatine in muscle to produce adenosine triphosphate (ATP), the body's energy molecule. Total creatine kinase measurement in serum has remained the best overall marker for detection and monitoring of skeletal and muscle stress.[37] Injury or diseases to striated muscle most commonly cause increases in total serum creatine kinase. In this case, colostrum reduced createine kinase levels.

Improved Sports Performance Among Power Athletes In another double blind, placebo controlled trial from the University of South Australia, 51 male power sport participants completed an eight-week standardized training program while consuming 60 grams daily of either colostrum or whey protein.[38] The athletes were tested for power performance in a battery of tests before beginning supplementation and at weeks four and eight. The subjects followed dietary guidelines and food diaries were kept throughout the trial. No additional supplementation was allowed. The colostrum group significantly improved their maximal vertical jump heights compared to the whey protein group. The colostrum group also improved their post-recovery vertical jump performance significantly more than the control group. There were strong trends for the colostrum group towards greater improvements than the control group in absolute and relative peak power outputs in cycling and peak force generated by knee flexion exercises.

Improved Performance Among Women Elite Athletes In a double-blind placebo controlled study, the effect of colostrum on rowing performance was studied in a group of elite female rowers. Eight female rowers from the South Australian Sports Institute completed a nine-week training program while consuming 60 grams per day of bovine colostrum powder or whey protein powder. All subjects consumed their normal diets and kept food diaries throughout the study period. There were significantly greater increases in the distance covered and work done by week nine. Buffer capacity was also higher in the colostrum group. These results indicate that oral supplementation with bovine colostrum improves rowing performance in elite female rowers, said the researchers.

HOW COLOSTRUM HELPS

Growth factors contained in colostrum stimulate faster rapid repair of damaged tissues.

One factor is reduction in muscle damage as indicated by changes in creatine kinase (CK) activity. Athletes receiving colostrum tend to show less muscle damage. Colostrum benefits may also be due to improvement in protein synthesis, since researchers noted a greater increase in thigh girth in the colostrum group.

With consistent use, the growth factors in colostrum continually regenerate and rebuild the entire body.

And even if you're not the athletic type, you can still take advantage of the muscle building and metabolic benefits that are found in colostrum. The same factors which are so sought-after by athletes can contribute to weight loss and the building of lean muscle. They produce a toning and tightening effect throughout the entire body and they can make a big difference when it comes to the ability to repair and regenerate new tissue. Studies have shown that levels of IGF-1 decrease with age but by supplementing with colostrum, the ravages of age and exercise are much less severe.

LEMON ALMOND BUTTER

Blend Colostrum6 and lemon juice until smooth and creamy. Add in the almond butter and Barlean's Lemon Swirl. Note that the mixture takes on a new thickness. Add more lemon juice if needed. This mixture is fabulous with apples and other fruits. Take an extra step and grate a whole apple and then mix in the Lemon Almond Butter in with it. Refreshing and juicy!

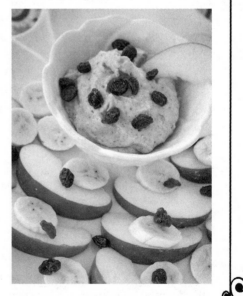

1 T	Immune-Tree Colostrum6
¼ t	fresh lemon juice
4 T	almond butter
2 T	Barlean's Lemon Swirl

13

⚜

ANTI-AGING

I t is documented that hormones in the body decrease as we age. Studies indicate advanced age is associated with reduced levels of GH and its counterpart, IGF-I. It has been reported that by the age of 40, the concentration of IGF-I is less than half of what it was at age 20. Likewise, GH decreases about 80 percent between the ages of 21 and 61. Hormone reductions cause the skin to thin and dry out, muscle mass and bone density to decrease, cholesterol levels to rise, cardiovascular function to weaken and mental abilities to decline.

In a study in the *New England Journal of Medicine*, 6 months of GH treatment not only stopped the body from aging, but actually reversed the effects of years of hormone deficiency. This study, conducted with 26 men between the ages of 61 and 80, resulted in an overall decrease in body fat (up to 14 percent), an increase in lean muscle mass and thicker, more elastic skin. The study equated these changes with the reversal of 10 to 20 years of aging!

Growth hormones are being used on an increasing basis to prevent aging. Colostrum supplementation, compared to hormone replacement, may be a desirable option. The most compelling evidence in favor of colostrum is that it is a "food" and won't have some potentially serious side effects from the use of hGH injections. Colostrum is 100 percent pure, providing only substances that the body can use. There are no side effects and thousands of years of use have proved there are no complications.

The other obvious benefit is that it is balanced and complete. It contains all the hormones used by the body—not just one—and in appropriate proportions. In colostrum, these growth hormones are accompanied with all the factors and co-factors to work together for maximum benefit. The more we learn about the body, the more we understand that no function is completely independent. Furnishing a "whole food" is usually much preferred over supplying portions in isolation.

Besides having more energy, those who use colostrum regularly report that they just feel better. GH affects neurotransmitters in the brain, improving mood and enhancing mental functions and memory. "I have also noticed that my outlook on life is more positive," writes colostrum user Ronald O.

"After two years of taking colostrum, I ran into a friend I hadn't seen in a couple of years," says Mary P. "The following week he called me and asked me what I had been doing to look so young. He said I looked 10 years younger than when he had seen me last —that my skin was visibly different."

Growth factors also stimulate cell growth in the dermal layer of the skin, improving both skin thickness and elasticity. Wrinkles are reduced and the skin takes on a soft texture. Cell proliferation is also stimulated in the scalp and some colostrum users report hair regrowth.

Here's hair growth recipe to try: "I decided to make a topical formula for my skin," says Dorothy H. "I mixed colostrum with extra virgin olive oil and put it on my face at night. Believe it or not, there is hair growing from the places in my hairline where it had begun to get thin."

"I have a lot of patients who love colostrum for the anti-aging effects," says Greg Barsten, DC, CCSP, CCN "I treated a naturopath recently for low energy by using colostrum. Not only did her energy pick up but her husband (an engineer of the skeptical nature) came to me wanting some. 'Just look at her face—the wrinkles are gone!' he said. I have had several people come to me asking for colostrum because of what it has done for their friends."

HOW TO USE

Combine first-milking colostrum with laminaria seaweed (limu), the antioxidant fucoidan, zeolite and acety l-carnitine (ALC).

The zeolite is to aid the detoxification processes. After the Chernobyl nuclear disaster, people in the affected regions were given a food product containing zeolite to absorb the radioactive fallout, and livestock in Scandinavia and Scotland that ate the product excreted radio isotopes more quickly. In the March-April 2003 issue of Anticancer Research, researchers from the RuÄ'er BoškoviÄ‡ Institute, Division of Molecular Medicine, in Bijenicka Zagreb, Croatia, reported that "treatment with micronized zeolite clinoptilolite (MZ) led to improvement of the overall health status, prolongation of lifespan and decrease of tumor size in some cases."

Many studies have shown that ALC aids cognitive health and depression. ALC is a neuroprotective agent because of the following properties: (a) antioxidant action; (b) mitochondrial energy supply; (c) membrane stability function; and (d) nerve impulse transmission enhancement.

Limu is a brown seaweed. These edible seaweeds contain large quantities of fucoidan fiber to absorb fat soluble toxins that are released into the bloodstream during weight-loss periods. This was shown in a 2002 study from the Journal of Agricultural and Food Chemistry where researchers report "that the administration of seaweed... is efficient in preventing the absorption and reabsorption of dioxin from the gastrointestinal tract and might be useful in treatment of humans exposed to dioxin." Brown seaweed supplies iodine to regulate the thyroid and has been studied for its effect on weight loss, especially abdominal tissue. Brown seaweed's anti-aging effect is against genetic damage to the cells.

An effervescent and isotonic rescue powder for quick absorption is available that has the same electrolyte balance as the blood and is highly absorbable with immediate delivery into the system because it bypasses the digestive process.

We're all searching for true super foods. The anti-aging properties of colostrum, with its growth and immune regulation factors, can be used effectively for cell renewal, muscle repair and longevity.

COCO PEACH PIE

So many of us today want something rich, creamy and sweet, but we don't want gluten or excessive carbs. Coco Peach Pie made with coconut milk and first-milking colostrum is without the sugar and the crust. This recipe can be used for a pie filling or just a luscious adventure all on its own.

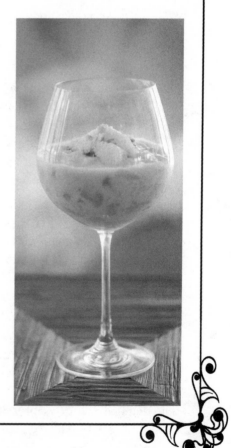

Combine peaches, coconut milk, ginger, lime, colostrum, XyloSweet, salt and spices in a sauce-pan. Bring to a simmer and let cook until peaches are soft. Mix arrowroot with the water and add to the mixture. Cook for a few minutes until the mixture thickens. Remove from the heat and serve or chill to serve cold. Top with coconut flakes, walnuts or anything else your heart desires!

2 C	fresh peaches (chopped)
1 C	coconut milk
1 t	grated ginger
1	lime (juiced)
3 t+	XyloSweet
1 ½ T	arrowroot
3 T	water
1-2 T	Immune-Tree Colostrum6 (optional)
	pinch of salt
	pinches of clove and/or nutmeg (optional)

SHOPPING FOR COLOSTRUM

Despite the many claims made by manufacturers, all bovine colostrum products are not the same. There is a wide variation in the composition of products on the market. Manufacturers use everything from whey protein to true, first-milking, complete colostrum, and unfortunately, they are all being marketed as "colostrum." It is very difficult for the average consumer to find a quality product, which matches its claims, without trying brand after brand. This chapter identifies some of the major differences between colostrum products currently on the market and puts the reader in a position to make an educated choice.

The most obvious considerations in choosing high quality bovine colostrum are those that have been discussed throughout this book, including the following:

- Is it true colostrum? Has it been collected as soon as possible (no later than 8 hours) after the birth of the calf?
- Is it complete colostrum? Have any of the components, such as the lipids, been removed or altered?
- Is the product manufactured so as to protect the biological activity of all of the components?
- Is it guaranteed free of hormones, antibiotics, pesticides and harmful bacteria?

THE DAIRY HERD

There are other questions to be considered which relate to the cows themselves. Are they healthy? How are they cared for? What do they eat? How many cows contribute to the colostrum in the product? Answers to these questions should help you determine whether or not you are buying high quality colostrum.

Companies marketing the highest quality bovine colostrum usually have access to at least 500 dairy herds, averaging about 300 cows each. All of these animals must meet Grade A standards for milk and they must be given a nutritionally sound, controlled diet, both line- and pasture-fed. Since cows probably will not all have the same levels of biologically active components in their individual colostrum, collecting from a large number of animals in different herds and "pooling" their colostrum, assures a uniform, maximum level of all of the beneficial components.

Similarly, the use of a large number of cows from many herds also assures *antibody diversity* in each production lot. As we've discussed, antibodies in colostrum are a result of the mother's immune response to foreign substances. These foreign substances include the various vaccines administered to protect the animal, and a variety of infectious organisms, which she has been exposed to throughout her life. Obviously, not every cow will be exposed to exactly the same pathogens, so colostrum that comes from many cows on many different dairy farms will have greater antibody diversity.

Antibody diversity is not a benefit of strict open pasturing, however. Some manufacturers claim that open pasturing produces more antibodies because of the exposure to more soil-borne organisms. In fact, most soil-borne organisms (other than those from animal excrement) are not "infectious" to cows. If simple soil-borne organisms caused infections in cows, they would be sickly all the time. These organisms are also not infectious to humans and the presence of their antibodies in the colostrum provides no actual health benefit.

Many years ago, US dairy farmers recognized that open pasturing of dairy cows, including breeding and unsupported calf delivery in the pasture environment, could actually cause several serious problems. It led to a higher incidence of disease, negatively affected milk production volumes and the quality of milk and had an adverse effect of the health of the calves, because there was no way to assure that they received an adequate amount of colostrum. It has become a dairy industry standard in the United States that all pregnant cows due to deliver, are monitored around the clock. Most dairy farms have a maternity ward away from the main herd for this purpose. This system, as opposed to dropping calves in the open pasture, prevents disease, facilitates better calf handing and allows for quicker, cleaner collection of colostrum.

Another consideration in regard to the dairy herd is that not every mother cow provides high quality colostrum. Studies show that only those cows that have experienced three or more live births produce colostrum with a maximum amount of bioactive substances and a sufficient quantity and diversity of antibodies to be considered "high quality."

COLLECTION

The United States Department of Agriculture defines colostrum as the "milk" collected in the first six milkings after birth. This was done to keep colostrum out of the milk intended for human consumption. We now know that bovine colostrum formation ceases at birth, and that true undiluted colostrum can only be obtained during the first milking, which must take place within a few hours after the birth of the calf.

Some manufacturers still use the original USDA classification of colostrum to justify the sale of mislabeled products from multiple milkings after the birth of the calf. This obviously results in much more "product" per cow, but the colostrum is significantly diluted, dramatically diminishing its potency and effectiveness as a supplement. This "colostrum" can never provide the same range of benefits that can be experienced with high quality first milking colostrum.

PROCESSING

Once colostrum is collected, it should be frozen immediately. Then the frozen colostrum is transferred, as quickly as possible, to the processing facility. This is very important since no milk product is completely free of bacteria. Leaving the colostrum in the liquid state would encourage spoilage and bacteria growth.

Some colostrum manufacturers claim that freezing destroys the biologically active components, making then insoluble and difficult for the body to absorb. There is simply no scientific evidence to support these claims. Proper freezing does not alter the water-soluble nature of organic substances. In fact, laboratories constantly freeze protein solutions in order to store these molecules while still maintaining their biological activity. Science has established that the method for thawing, rather than freezing, can denature proteins. To avoid this, the protein solution must be thawed slowly at a temperature that does not exceed human body temperature, 98.6 F. (37 C.).

COMPLETE COLOSTRUM

Colostrum provides the best physical "start" a newborn could have. This "start" is not medically adjusted, strained or rearranged in any way.

Instead, it goes directly from the mother to the newborn. It is ridiculous to imagine adding steps to this natural process to change the colostrum before feeding it to the newborn. And yet that is just what many manufacturers do with bovine colostrum intended for human use.

In order to experience all the benefits from colostrum, it should not only meet the collection and processing criteria mentioned above, but it must also be complete colostrum. A complete colostrum is one that has not had any components removed, or any other substance added that could change colostrum's characteristics, alter the balance of biologically active components or interfere with their effectiveness.

Some companies that market "colostrum," physically or chemically remove components like the fat. This changes the composition of the colostrum, interfering with the relationships of the active components, and even removing other valuable ingredients. Manufacturers argue that removing the fat increases the shelf life of the product. This argument is simply without scientific merit. Rancidity in dairy products is only associated with fluid materials and is not a consideration for a properly dried colostrum powder.

Rather than improving the product, fat removal has several negative consequences. As we've talked about before, several vitamins and growth factors are so closely associated with the fat in colostrum that when it is removed, these valuable components are also removed. Equally important, is the role that the fat plays in helping the body effectively use various colostral components. For example, when complete colostrum enters the stomach, enzymes there act upon the casein and fat to form a cheese-like curd, which protects the active components, keeping them from breaking down in the stomach. This helps to assure that as much of each biologically active component as possible reaches the small intestine where absorption into the bloodstream occurs.

CHEMICAL COMPOSITION

Colostral fat is important for another reason. The amounts of fat, protein and lactose in powdered colostrum are excellent markers to identify it as a high quality product. When these amounts are out of proportion, it is an indicator that either the product is diluted with "transitional milk," or some components have been removed during processing.

In the chart below, we have the actual findings from studies done at a major dairy product-testing laboratory comparing the amounts of key ingredients in true bovine colostrum to what is present in "colostrum" products on the

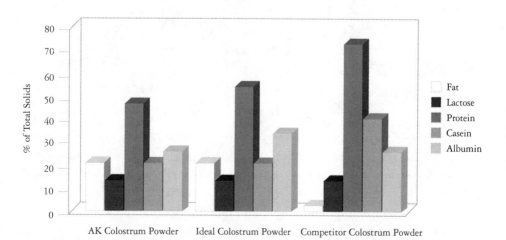

market. The *Ideal Colostrum Powder* in the middle of the chart was carefully prepared and made from a large pool of colostrum, collected within six hours after birth. The results of the tests clearly demonstrate the differences between these products. The colostrum powder on the left is virtually identical in chemical composition to the ideal colostrum powder. In sharp contrast, the colostrum powder on the right has had most of the fat removed and the relationship between the remaining components has been dramatically altered.

Does this really mean that one product would provide less health benefits than the other? To answer that question, refer to the graph below, which compares amounts of IGF-1 in a complete colostrum versus that in widely marketed products. These studies were performed by the Endocrinology Laboratory of a major U.S. college of veterinary medicine. Three production lots were tested to verify the findings. As you can see, only one product even comes close to having the amount of IGF-1 found in a complete, first milking colostrum. Since IGF-1 is one of the most influential components of colostrum, a product with less IGF-1 simply may not be able to produce all the health benefits we've discussed in this book.

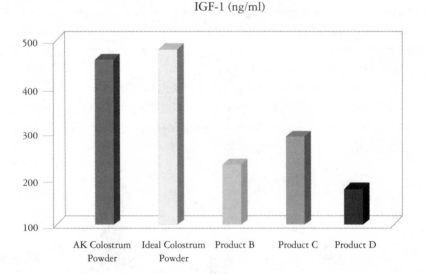

IGF-1 (ng/ml)

Unfortunately, these aren't tests you can conduct in your kitchen at home. But every manufacturer of colostrum has to know the fat, protein and lactose content of their product in order to control the manufacturing process. Asking for these figures and comparing them will give you a good idea of the quality of the product.

ORGANIC STATUS

Another question to ask is whether or not the product has been tested and found to be completely free of hormones, antibiotics and pesticides. If you're taking a product to improve your health, be sure there is nothing in it that may actually compromise your well being. Only the finest quality colostrum products can claim to "test organic" and be guaranteed free of these substances.

MAKING THE CHOICE

The best way to apply the above knowledge in choosing a brand of colostrum is to ask a lot of questions. If a company can't or won't answer the following questions, then keep looking for one that gives you sufficient information to feel confident that you're getting the best possible product

The following are some things you want to know:

- Is the colostrum collected from Grade A, certified dairy cows and are the cows maintained in a healthy, controlled environment?
- Is there a time limit after birth during which all of the colostrum is collected and what is that time limit?
- Is the colostrum complete? Has anything been added or removed, other than the moisture?
- What kind of testing do you do to assure that this colostrum is biologically active?
- Can you show me evidence of the composition of this colostrum, particularly in terms of the amount of fat, protein and lactose?
- Has this colostrum been tested and declared free of hormones, antibiotics and pesticides?

If you decide to be among the thousands of health conscious consumers who are benefiting from the use of colostrum, make sure you find the very best and be certain that it is high quality first-milking complete colostrum.

RICH CHERRY CHOCOLATE SUPREME

Combine all ingredients and blend until creamy and frothy. If you are a chocolate lover, this smoothie will rock your soul. The flavor is rich with substance that will fuel, satisfy and please you. For an extra treat, garnish both smoothies with fresh mint!

1	scoop MHP Paleo Protein Triple Chocolate
1/3 C	hemp seeds
1 T	soy lecithin granules
1 T	Immune-Tree Colostrum6
½ to ¾ C	frozen cherries
	water
2 C	ice

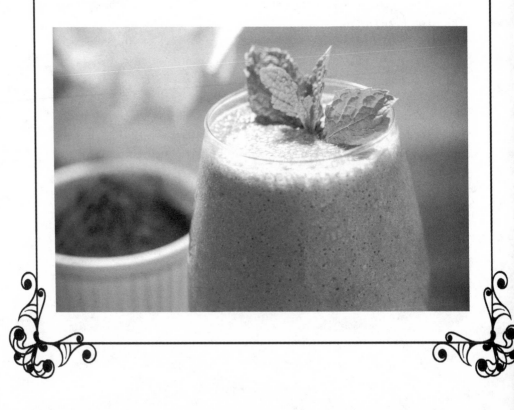

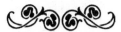

COLOSTRUM BACKGROUND
Colostrum FAQs

What is colostrum?

Those of us who are really in the know don't think of colostrum as a dietary supplement. It certainly isn't the same as an herb or isolated vitamin or mineral. Rather, colostrum is a whole food pre-milk fluid concentrate, replete with thousands of health-promoting, disease-fighting nutrients. Many haven't even been identified or characterized yet.

What does colostrum contain that makes it so powerful a health aide?

Colostrum is every newborn's "first food." It is the perfectly balanced "first meal" that every mammal gives its newborn. It is produced by the mother for only a short period of time; yet, it contains numerous compounds which stimulate and support many processes in the body, including activation of the immune system, regeneration and repair of tissues and growth of *all* types of cells.

Complete, first milking bovine colostrum primarily contains proteins, with its other main ingredients being fat and lactose (milk sugar). The chart below shows how the relationship of these three major components changes with time.

Protein

Many of the ingredients in colostrum responsible for the growth and immune benefits are biologically active proteins.

COMPOSITION OF LIQUID BOVINE COLOSTRUM

Hrs. After Calving	Total % Protein	Total % Fat	Total % Lactose	Total % Solids
0	17.57	5.10	2.19	26.99
6	10.00	6.85	2.71	20.46
12	6.05	3.80	3.71	14.53
24	4.52	3.40	3.98	12.77
36	3.98	3.55	3.97	12.22
48	3.74	2.80	3.97	11.46

Fat

The fat in colostrum is one of its most underrated and misunderstood components. There are various opinions about colostral fat, many negative. Some say the fat serves no purpose at all. Others claim that its presence in dried colostrum leads to faster deterioration of the product. Both of these arguments are simply untrue. In fact, one company that removes the fat from "colostrum" later adds a component of the fat back to their product. They add this component to make the product more digestible, which is one of the functions of the fat in the first place.

The digestive aid that colostral fat provides is one of its most important benefits. For example, colostral fat is necessary to digest the protein casein, a major protein in both colostrum and milk that aids in calcium absorption. Casein is digested by forming a cottage cheeselike curd through enzyme action in the stomach. Colostral fat is the basis for the curd and without it most of the nutritional value of the casein is lost. This is just one example of the benefits of fat found in colostrum. Again, referring to the chart, you'll notice that the colostral fat content increases with time. One reason for this increase is to support the digestion of increasing amounts of casein.

The fat in colostrum also plays an important role in delivering some of the biologically active substances to the body. The following components are associated so closely with fat that they are removed if colostrum is de-fatted—a common practice in colostrum processing:

- Vitamins A, D, E and K
- Steroid hormones and corticosteroids (the tiny amounts in colostrum are extremely effective in reducing inflammation associated with tissue trauma and infection)
- Some growth factors (notably IGF-1)
- Insulin

Lactose (milk sugar)

The third major ingredient, lactose, makes up 8-13% of *complete, first milking* colostrum solids. Lactose is an immediate source of energy when it is broken down to glucose and galactose by lactase, an enzyme in the saliva and stomach. As you can see from the chart, the amount of lactose in colostrum increases significantly during the first days of a calf's life, as the newborn's energy demands increase.

The lactose in colostrum can also act as an energy source for humans, since most of us have lactase in our saliva and digestive system. However, there are individuals whose bodies produce too little of the lactase enzyme or none at all. These people are said to be "lactose intolerant" because lactose does not break down in the digestive tract. Instead, it can cause bloating and discomfort.

But there is hope, even for the lactose intolerant. As shown in the previous chart, the amount of lactose in *first milking* colostrum—collected in the first six to eight hours—is about one-half of what it is at twelve hours. At 24 hours, it is almost three times the original amount. A first-milking colostrum contains enough lactose to improve energy levels but not so much as to cause many of the possible discomforts associated with lactose intolerance. In addition, other ingredients in colostrum can heal the intestinal wall, reducing or eliminating many food allergies—including all reactions to dairy products. This means that, for many colostrum users, lactose intolerance is now only a thing of the past.

What is the difference between colostrum and regular cow's milk?

So far we've focused on the changing levels of proteins, fat and lactose as colostrum transitions to milk. Vitamin and mineral levels also change, creating a striking difference between colostrum, first milk and the milk that you might find at your grocery store. The following comparative facts about colostrum and milk provide even further evidence as to the benefits a complete first milking colostrum can provide.

Colostrum contains 10 times more vitamin A than milk, 3 times more vitamin D than milk, at least 10 times more iron than milk and more calcium, phosphorous and magnesium than milk.

The immune factors in colostrum provide protection for the newborn against bacteria, toxins, virus and disease. They activate numerous processes which are critical to the healthy function of the immune system. They stimulate factors that heighten the overall immune response and provide support to a developing immune system until it is ready to function on its own. These same factors offer similar benefits to adults and children—stimulating and supporting weakened immune functions, while, paradoxically quieting an overactive immune system.

Many people have been impressed with the potential for "passive immunity" from colostrum for protection from bacteria and viral pathogens. And although there is some immunity "passed on" from colostrum to recipient, other immune factors in colostrum strengthen the overall immune response. In the long run, this also has far-reaching health benefits. It means that a weakened immune system can be strengthened to the point where it can "ward off" invading organisms on its own. This is the ultimate benefit, and the way the immune system was meant to function—without the assistance of donated antibodies via inoculation or otherwise.

When you think about it, that's what we all want—a healthy immune system which is capable of taking care of anything that comes along. With a healthy immune system we would not have to rely on vaccines and flu shots, which have their drawbacks and are certainly not 100 percent effective. The immune factors in colostrum build and support *all* the processes which relate to healthy immune function. With the regular addition of colostrum to the diet, most individuals report a heightened immune response—fewer colds, flu, and allergies. They also notice that when they do catch a cold, they are able to move through it much more easily.

Growth factors contained in colostrum are instrumental in promoting rapid healing and repair of damaged tissues in the newborn. They are instrumental in facilitating normal growth and they work with the immune factors to support processes throughout the entire body. For adults and children, these same growth factors are involved in the healing and repair of all types of tissues and organs. With consistent use, they continually regenerate and rebuild the entire body. As with the components of any "food," the growth factors in colostrum typically "go" where they are needed—sealing the lining of the intestinal tract, repairing damaged muscle tissue (including the heart), healing wounds and rebuilding organs and tissues.

Many of the effects of the growth factors are considered "anti-aging." The youthful "side effects" of taking colostrum include, more energy, elevated moods, smoother skin, wrinkle reduction, better digestion, balancing of blood sugar levels and weight loss, to name a few.

For how long has bovine colostrum been consumed by humans?

For thousands of years, Ayurvedic physicians and sacred healers known as Rishis, have used bovine (cow) colostrum for medicinal purposes—for everything from immune deficiencies and age-related symptoms to treatment of the common cold. Even today, colostrum is delivered with the milk in some parts of India.

In the Scandinavian countries, colostrum has been used in folk medicine for centuries. The birth of a calf is celebrated and the colostrum is used in the making of a dessert to promote good health. As early as 1799, Dr. Hufland researched the benefits of colostrum on the health and growth of newborn cattle. His studies laid the groundwork for the early medicinal use of colostrum.

Colostrum was used worldwide prior to World War II. It was known and respected for its immune-boosting capabilities and was extensively used in the treatment of rheumatoid arthritis in the 1950s. In the United States, it was used for its antibiotic properties before antibiotics were available.

In 1962, Albert Sabin developed a successful polio vaccine from isolated antibodies found in bovine colostrum. With the technology that erupted during the aftermath of World War II came penicillin and the sulfa drugs. These new drugs worked so quickly that many traditional methods were forgotten in favor of faster-working antibiotics.

With our current arsenal of antibiotics and other drugs, why should we go 'back in time' and ingest colostrum?

Now, after 50 years of antibiotic use, we are seeing some serious drawbacks. Their overuse has caused resistant strains of bacteria requiring stronger and stronger antibiotics which in turn can trigger unhealthy side effects. So, like many other things, we have come full circle and we are again beginning to consider the older, more traditional remedies that were used for centuries before fullscale reliance upon antibiotics and other drugs.

Do colostrum's uses go beyond the field of human health?

As with many of the remedies which are resurfacing, the veterinary industry leads the way. This is the case with colostrum which has been utilized in the animal industry for many years. Dr. Richard Cockrum began experimenting with colostrum over 30 years ago. As a young veterinary student, he observed the rapid decline in the health of animals which were deprived of colostrum. His research resulted in the development of a complete line of veterinary colostrum formulations which are still used worldwide— often in place of antibiotics. His work has paved the way in the development of processing methods which ensure safety while retaining the biological activity of the delicate components in colostrum.

Have any scientific studies been published on colostrum's health benefits?

During the last 20 years, the scientific community has rediscovered the multitude of benefits from this "food." Over 10,000 experimental and clinical studies have been published on the use of colostrum and its components to treat a variety of diseases and health concerns. In fact, pharmaceutical companies have been so intrigued with many of the components in colostrum, that they have synthesized (genetically engineered) several of them, including interferon, protease inhibitors, gamma globulin, growth hormone and insulinlike growth factor-I. The latter has been used in expensive anti-aging clinics for 10 to 15 years.

How is bovine colostrum obtained?

Bovine colostrum is produced before birth and can be taken only for a short period of time without being diluted by the subsequent production of milk. At the time of birth, potency is at its peak. The active elements, including immune factors, growth factors, antioxidants and anti-inflammatory agents, are at their highest concentrations. However, in less than 12 hours, the concentration of these components is only half of what it was at the time of birth. This makes colostrum a limited commodity; yet, because of the extensive dairy industry, sufficient quantities are available for human use as a dietary supplement.

Why bovine colostrum?

There are several reasons why bovine colostrum is the chosen source for human supplementation.

Other than the actual antibodies, (specifically produced as a result of contact with pathogens), most of the immune factors and growth factors contained in bovine colostrum have been identified in human colostrum and shown to be very similar. Not only are they very similar, but some of them are many times more potent. For this reason, when it comes to healing and regeneration, bovine colostrum may even be better than human colostrum.

Bovine colostrum is not species specific and any mammal can benefit from its use. For this reason, bovine colostrum has been used successfully for many years on a wide variety of animal species. Bovine colostrum is like the universal blood type, "O," which can be utilized by any other blood type. Studies indicate that all mammalian species, including man, can benefit from bovine colostrum.

Cows produce an abundance of this "first food"—enough to supply human needs without depriving newborn calves. Most cows produce between 2 and 2 ½ gallons of colostrum from the first milking. Calves need only about two quarts.

The dairy industry in this country is perfectly suited for the sanitary removal and processing of bovine colostrum. In addition, because the dairy industry is so large, there are plenty of dairy cows from which to "pool" colostrum.

But isn't the newborn calf deprived of an important food for its health?

The first thing most people want to know is: "What happens to the poor calf? Does it have *its first meal* taken away?" Fortunately, for everyone, a cow produces more than enough colostrum. If a calf were left to suckle its mother, it would consume only about one of the two quarts of colostrum it typically requires, then lie down to rest. While the calf is sleeping, precious biological factors would be reabsorbed back into the mother and lost forever. For this reason, it has been standard practice for many years to remove the colostrum from a mother cow and feed it to the calf from a bottle at intervals so that it can receive the full benefit of this "first milk." Calves actually get more of the benefits of colostrum this way and are healthier with a lower mortality rate.

Research has also shown that there is a point at which calves receive no further benefit from additional colostrum. Two quarts is usually sufficient unless there are complications. The rest of the colostrum has been used in the veterinary industry for years. Remember, cow colostrum can be helpful for all mammalian species. Rest assured, no dairy farmer would allow a newborn calf to go without colostrum. In most cases, it would mean certain death since cows rely completely on colostrum for their immunity.

How do cows make colostrum?

Colostrogenesis, which is the formation of colostrum, and lactogenesis, the formation of milk, are completely separate processes. They are each controlled by specific hormonal changes and influenced by different physical factors. A common misunderstanding about bovine colostrum is in thinking that it continues to be produced after the calf is born. This is not the case. The hormonal changes that occur at the time of birth cause colostrum production to cease in the mother cow. This is perhaps the *single most important thing* to understand when it comes to colostrum quality.

During the last five to seven years, dairy science has developed a deeper understanding of what bovine colostrum actually is and how it is formed. Numerous studies have now shown that colostrum formation in the cow begins several weeks prior to birth, accelerates as parturition nears and ceases upon the birth of the calf.

So, let's take a closer look at the process:

The formation of colostrum is initiated in the cow three to four weeks before the birth. At this time, growth factors and other transforming substances are released which influence the appearance of receptors on the lining of the mammary gland. These receptors facilitate the transfer of materials from the mother's blood into the gland.

Two weeks before birth, these receptors become fully active. Antibodies, known as immunoglobulins, from the mother's blood attach to the receptors and are transferred into the mammary gland. Additional receptors transport other substances prior to birth.

About two days before birth, the hormonal balance shifts, initiating the production of secretions and switching on the ability of cells in the mammary tissue to synthesize numerous substances. At the time of birth, the mammary gland is filled with a mixture of immune factors, growth factors, nucleotides, vitamins, enzymes and minerals which are perfectly balanced to activate and support over 50 processes in the newborn calf.

What are the similarities and differences between human and bovine colostrum?
The majority of human immunity is transferred through the placenta. Babies are born with a certain amount of immunity—colostrum is desirable but not absolutely necessary for a baby's survival. Cows receive *no* immunity through the placenta and their immune system is *completely dependent* upon the receipt of colostrum immediately after birth. For this reason, the concentration of antibodies or immunoglobulins is much higher in bovine than in human colostrum. A 1979 study revealed that the immunoglobulin portion of bovine colostrum is 86 percent IgG—the most important immunoglobulin in the body. Human colostrum contains only two percent IgG. Other biological factors are also more concentrated in bovine colostrum.

Bovine colostrum has a higher concentration of growth factors. These growth factors (mainly IGF-I and GH) are involved in repair and rejuvenation in the human system. The higher growth factor concentration in bovine colostrum is ideal for building lean muscle, repair of damaged tissues due to age or injury, balancing blood sugar levels, reducing wrinkles, increasing energy, and a lot of other benefits. For the adult who is seeking healing, muscle tone, rejuvenation and/or anti-aging effects, bovine colostrum is even more promising than human colostrum would be—if it were even an option.

On the other hand, many of the key components in bovine colostrum have been shown to be very similar to those contained in human colostrum. In fact, many references refer to them as being identical. Although complete identity is an overstatement, bovine colostrum contains many very similar components which appear to benefit the human body in the same way as those similar components from human colostrum. For example, the important growth factor, IGF-I, found in bovine colostrum, contains the identical amino acid sequence except for a short segment on the front of the bovine molecule. This gets split off during digestion in the stomach, leaving an identical version of the human molecule. Other important biological factors are either identical or so similar that they function in a like manner.

Is the production of colostrum by humans the same as that in cows?
Colostrogenesis is somewhat different in the human system. A human mother will continue to produce colostrum for about two days. This has caused many to assume that the bovine process is the same. However, bovine colostrum production *ceases* at the time of birth. Hormonal changes associated with birth block any further transfer of substances from the mother's blood into the mammary gland. Therefore, the substance available at the time of birth is the only true colostrum. It has a composition characterized by:

A high protein content—mostly the Immunoglobulin G (IgG, a class of antibodies).

- High concentrations of growth promoters.
- Low lactose concentrations (a milk sugar).
- Milk fat concentrations between 8-13%.
- Why do so many health experts talk about first-milking colostrum?

At birth, when the placenta is eliminated, the level of the hormone called progesterone, falls dramatically. Simultaneously, a protein-based substance develops in the lining of the mammary gland which blocks any further transfer of substances from the mother's blood. These changes, along with the physical removal of the colostrum, signal the production of milk—referred to as lactogenesis.

At the time of birth, almost all of the biologically active components present in the udder are transferred from the circulation of the mother, while most substances found in later fluids are produced by cells within the udder itself. These factors, combined with the time of collection after birth, play a major role in establishing the quality of bovine colostrum, which is really a golden color. Removal of even a small quantity of colostrum immediately after birth, as would occur via suckling, results in a very substantial influx of a different fluid produced by the cells in the udder, known as transitional milk, markedly diluting the true colostrum. In addition, if the true colostrum is not removed from the udder during the first 6-8 hours after birth of the calf, the mother's system begins to reabsorb the biologically active components back into her circulation. Therefore, the only colostrum that contains all of the biologically active components in the appropriate proportions is that which is obtained at the first milking within 6 hours after birth. Major American dairy producers are keenly aware of this and most maintain maternity wards, separate from the main herd, to support the birth of their calves. They no longer allow the calf to suckle, but, rather, collect the complete colostrum within hours after birth and feed an adequate quantity to the calf via a nursing bottle.

The removal of even small amounts of colostrum triggers the production of a significant quantity of milk. If colostrum is not removed, or is only partially removed, the mother's system will begin to reabsorb many of the biologically active substances within six to eight hours. This is why most dairy farmers "milk" the cow and feed the required amount back to the calf. For those of us who are interested in the best quality colostrum, the *first milking* is the only time it can be obtained in an undiluted state and before biological factors begin to be reabsorbed into the mother. This assures that it is still high in the immune and growth factors which are of interest to us.

Misunderstanding the shift from production of colostrum to production of milk has caused many to believe that good quality colostrum can be produced and collected from the first five milkings of the cow. This is not the case. In order to illustrate the significance of timing vs. quality, let's examine something called the 80/20 rule.

The 80/20 rule is an accepted concept in dairy science. It refers to the fact that when a cow is milked, no more than 80 percent of the contents of the mammary glands can be removed without damage to the cow. This being the case, the *first milking* of the cow after she gives birth, contains 80 percent of the total colostrum which has been produced. The first milking is a true, undiluted colostrum. Any subsequent milking contains less and less of the total colostrum. For example: The second milking contains 80 percent of the 20 percent which was not removed during the first milking (or about 16 percent of the total colostrum). Even though this second milking contains 16 percent colostrum, it is in a highly diluted state. The third milking contains 80 percent of the remaining 20 percent (or about 3 percent of the total colostrum). Any "colostrum" which is collected after the second milking is in such a diluted state that it can hardly be called colostrum, and in the dairy industry is referred to as *transitional milk*. This is actually very important. One of the things we've noticed in recent years is that many consumers purchase colostrum seeking to obtain the same healing powers documented in many clinical studies but they come away disappointed with their colostrum experience. That is because altogether too many so-called colostrum products being distributed today are not

COMPOSITION OF BOVINE COLOSTRUM & TRANSITIONAL MILK

Hrs. After Calving	Total % Protein	Total % Fat	Total % Lactose
0	17.57	5.10	2.19
6	10.00	6.85	2.71
12	6.05	3.80	3.71
24	4.52	3.40	3.98
30	4.01	4.90	4.27
36	3.98	3.55	3.97
48	3.74	2.80	3.97
72	3.86	3.10	4.37
96	3.76	2.80	4.72

Fundamentals of Dairy Chemistry 1988

colostrum but transitional milk. That's why later on in this book, we'll devote an entire chapter to showing shoppers how to be savvy colostrum consumers.

To make this point a little more emphatic, we've taken information from a standard dairy industry text. (See next page.)

Note how fast the total protein fraction of colostrum drops. Within hours, the total protein content is dramatically reduced and within three days is only half of what it was upon birth. This is significant because a good portion of the biological factors which are of interest in colostrum are large protein molecules. The rapid drop in this fraction is indicative of the transition to milk. Also note the rapid increase in lactose, which increases by more than fourfold. This is another very good indicator of the presence of milk.

It is not difficult to determine where to draw the line between true colostrum and what has been called transitional milk. At what point in time is colostrum no longer pure colostrum? One colostrum expert has noted:

"Bovine colostrum is produced during the few weeks prior to birth of the calf and, due to hormonal changes in the mother, its production stops at birth. Secretions collected at the first milking during the first 6-8 hour period after birth contain complete colostrum with all of the beneficial components intact. Removal of even some of the colostrum results in the release of a different material, known as transitional milk, that dilutes any colostrum still present and changes its composition."

Since colostrum is a limited commodity, it is easy to see why anyone would want to stretch the collection of this valuable substance.

This is why many widely advertised colostrum products on the market today *are obtained from the first five milkings—as much as 72 hours following the birth of the calf.* Such products, although widely sold and labeled as colostrum, are not true or complete colostrum. We really do need better labeling requirements when it comes to aiding shoppers to make smart choices about their nutritional supplements, including colostrum.

It is worth noting that researchers who use colostrum in clinical trials usually seek first milking colostrum because they recognize that potency and quality are diminished with time. Much of the research referenced in this book as well as all of the clinical reports and anecdotes are based on use of first-milking colostrum. To expect similar results with adulterated colostrum or transitional milk being marketed as colostrum would be unfair to both consumers seeking the health benefits of colostrum and to those producers of true first-milking colostrum.

CHAPTER REFERENCES

1   Cesarone MR, Belcaro G, Di Renzo A, Dugall M, Cacchio M, Ruffini I, Pellegrini L, Del Boccio G, Fano F, Ledda A, Bottari A, Ricci A, Stuard S, Vinciguerra G.Prevention of influenza episodes with colostrum compared with vaccination in healthy and high-risk cardiovascular subjects: the epidemiologic study in San Valentino. Clin Appl Thromb Hemost. 2007 Apr;13(2):130-6.

2   Belcaro G, Cesarone MR, Cornelli U, Pellegini L, Ledda A, Grossi MG, Dugall M, Ruffini I, Fano F, Ricci A, Stuard S, Luzzi R, Grossi MG, Hosoi M. Prevention of flu episodes with colostrum and Bifivir compared with vaccination: an epidemiological, registry study. Panminerva Med. 2010 Dec;52(4):269-75.

3   Mitra, A.K., et al. "Hyperimmune cow colostrum reduces diarrhea due to rotavirus: a double-blind, controlled clinical trial." Acta Paediatr, 1995;84(9):996-1001.

4   Kim, K., et al. "In vitro and in vivo neutralizing activity of human colostrum and milk against purified toxins A and B of Clostridium difficile." J Infectious Diseases, 1984;150(1):57-61.

5   See for example: "http://216.239.39.100/search?q=cache:Gml7vqrkN-wC:www.medinfo. ufl.edu/year2/mmid/bms5300/bugs/closdif.html+Clostridium+difficile+colostrum& hl=en&ie=UTF-8"

6   Chen HY, Mollstedt O, Tsai MH, Kreider RB1.Potential Clinical Applications of Multi-Functional Milk Proteins and Peptides in Cancer Management. Curr Med Chem. 2014 Feb 5. [Epub ahead of print]

7   An MJ1, Cheon JH, Kim SW, Park JJ, Moon CM, Han SY, Kim ES, Kim TI, Kim WH.Bovine colostrum inhibits nuclear factor kappaB-mediated proinflammatory cytokine expression in intestinal epithelial cells. Nutr Res. 2009 Apr;29(4):275-80. doi: 10.1016/j.nutres.2009.03.011.

8   Masuda C, Wanibuchi H, Sekine K, et al. Chemopreventive effects of bovine lactoferrin on N-butyl-N-(4-hydroxybutyl)nitrosamine-induced rat bladder carcinogenesis. Jpn J Cancer Res. 2000 Jun;91(6):582-8.

9   Raymond J Playford, Christopher E Macdonald and Wendy S Johnson Colostrum and milk-derived peptide growth factors for the treatment of gastrointestinal disorders American Journal of Clinical Nutrition, Vol. 72, No. 1, 5-14, July 2000

10 Hirano M, Iweakiri R, Fujimoto K, et al. Epidermal growth factor enhances repair of rat intestinal mucosa damaged after oral administration of methotrexate. J Gastroenterol 1995;30:169–76.[Medline]

11 Sonis ST, Lindquist L, Van Vugt A, et al. Prevention of chemotherapy-induced ulcerative mucositis by transforming growth factor beta 3. Cancer Res 1994;54:1135–8.[Abstract]

12 Howarth GS, Francis GL, Cool JC, Ballard RW, Read LC. Milk growth factors enriched from cheese whey ameliorate intestinal damage by methotrexate when administered orally to rats. J Nutr 1996;126:2519–30.[Medline]

13 Gordler NM, McGurk M, Aqual S, Prince M. The effect of EGF mouthwash on cytotoxic-induced oral ulceration. Am J Clin Oncol 1995;18:403–6.[Medline]

14 Raymond J Playford, Christopher E Macdonald and Wendy S Johnson Colostrum and milk-derived peptide growth factors for the treatment of gastrointestinal disorders American Journal of Clinical Nutrition, Vol. 72, No. 1, 5-14, July 2000

15 Ebina T, Sato A, Umezu K, Aso H, Ishida N, Seki H, Tsukamoto T, Takase S, Hoshi S, Ohta M. Treatment of multiple sclerosis with anti-measles cow colostrum. Med Microbiol Immunol. 1984;173(2):87-93.

16 Kramski M, Center RJ, Wheatley AK, Jacobson JC, Alexander MR, Rawlin G, Purcell DF.Hyperimmune bovine colostrum as a low-cost, large-scale source of antibodies with broad neutralizing activity for HIV-1 envelope with potential use in microbicides. Antimicrob Agents Chemother. 2012 Aug;56(8):4310-9. doi: 10.1128/AAC.00453-12. Epub 2012 Jun 4.

17 Kaducu FO, Okia SA, Upenytho G, Elfstrand L, Florén CH.Effect of bovine colostrum-based food supplement in the treatment of HIV-associated diarrhea in Northern Uganda: a randomized controlled trial. Indian J Gastroenterol. 2011 Dec;30(6):270-6. doi: 10.1007/s12664-011-0146-0. Epub 2011 Dec 13.

18 Florén CH, Chinenye S, Elfstrand L, Hagman C, Ihse I.ColoPlus, a new product based on bovine colostrum, alleviates HIV-associated diarrhea. Scand J Gastroenterol. 2006 Jun;41(6):682-6.

19 Kaducu FO, ibid.

20 Florén CH, ibid.

21 Friedman J, Alam SM, Shen X, Xia SM, Stewart S, Anasti K, Pollara J, Fouda GG, Yang G, Kelsoe G, Ferrari G, Tomaras GD, Haynes BF, Liao HX, Moody MA, Permar SR.Isolation of HIV-1-neutralizing mucosal monoclonal antibodies from human colostrum. PLoS One. 2012;7(5):e37648. doi: 10.1371/journal.pone.0037648. Epub 2012 May 18.

22 Kaducu FO, ibid.

23 Korhonen H, Marnila P, Gill HS. Bovine milk antibodies for health. Br J Nutr. 2000 Nov;84 Suppl 1:S135-46.

24 Kramski M, ibid.

25 Kramski M, Lichtfuss GF, Navis M, Isitman G, Wren L, Rawlin G, Center RJ, Jaworowski A, Kent SJ, Purcell DF.Anti-HIV-1 antibody-dependent cellular cytotoxicity mediated by hyperimmune bovine colostrum IgG. Eur J Immunol. 2012 Oct;42(10):2771-81. doi: 10.1002/eji.201242469. Epub 2012 Aug 28.

26 Hollander, D. "Intestinal permeability, leaky gut, and intestinal disorders." Curr Gastroenterol Rep, 1999;1(5):410-416.

27   Keshavarzian, A., et al. "Leaky gut in alcoholic cirrhosis: a possible mechanism for alcohol-induced liver damage." Am J Gastroenterol, 1999;94(1):200-207.

28   Schwarz, B. "[Intestinal ischemic reperfusion syndrome: pathophysiology, clinical significance, therapy]." Wien Klin Wochenschr, 1999;111(14):539-548.

29   Pinotti L, Rosi F. Leptin in bovine colostrum and milk. Horm Metab Res. 2006 ;38(2):89-93.

30   Preuss HG, DiFerdinando D, Bagchi M, Bagchi D.Citrus aurantium as a thermogenic, weight-reduction replacement for ephedra: an overview. J Med. 2002;33(1-4):247-264.

31   Lopez HL, Ziegenfuss TN, Hofheins JE, Habowski SM, Arent SM, Weir JP, Ferrando AA. Eight weeks of supplementation with a multi-ingredient weight loss product enhances body composition, reduces hip and waist girth, and increases energy levels in overweight men and women. J Int Soc Sports Nutr. 2013;10(1):22. doi: 10.1186/1550-2783-10-22.

32   Loimaranta, V., et al. "Effects of bovine immune and non-immune whey preparations on the composition and pH response of human dental plaque." Eur J Oral Sci, 1999;107(4):244-250.

33   Janusz M, Zabłocka A. Colostrinin: a proline-rich polypeptide complex of potential therapeutic interest. Cell Mol Biol (Noisy-le-grand). 2013 Nov 3;59(1):4-11.

34   Leszek J, Inglot AD, Janusz M, Lisowski J, Krukowska K, Georgiades JA. Arch Immunol Ther Exp (Warsz) 1999;47(6):377-85.

35   Mero, A., et al. "Effects of bovine colostrum supplementation on serum IGF-I, IgG, hormone, and saliva IgA during training." J Appl Physiol, 1997;83(4):144-1151.

36   Buckley, J., et al. "Effect of an oral bovine colostrum supplement (intact TM) on running performance." Abstract from: 1998 Australian Conference of Science and Medicine in Sport, Adelaide, South Australia, October 1998.

37   Wu, A.H. & Perryman, M.B. "Clinical applications of muscle enzymes and proteins." Curr Opin Rheumatol, 1992;4(6):815-820.

38   Buckley, J., et al. ""Oral supplementation with bovine colostrum (intact TM) increases vertical jump performance." Presented at 4th Annual Congress of the European College of Sports Science, Rome 14-17 July, 1999.

HEALTH PRACTITIONER'S GUIDE

SCIENTIFIC AND MEDICAL RESEARCH
Related To Bovine Colostrum

Its Relationship And Use

IN THE MAINTENANCE

OF

HEALTH

IN HUMANS

SELECTED PUBLISHED ABSTRACTS

TRUE BOVINE COLOSTRUM
For the Practitioner

INTRODUCTION

Colostrum is the first milk-like fluid yielded from the mammary glands of mammals after parturition and is intended for ingestion by the newborn during the first hours of life. In most mammals, such as humans, many of the biologically active substances essential to development and survival, such as growth promoting substances and immunoglobulins, cross the placental barrier and are transferred to the fetus *in utero*. In sharp contrast, in ungulates, particularly bovines, essentially none of these biologically active substances cross the placental barrier and, thus, must be acquired by the offspring through suckling during the early hours of its life.

There is a considerable body of scientific evidence showing that if a calf fails to receive an adequate quantity of high quality complete colostrum, it will be more vulnerable to pathogens in its environment and will not develop a proper body mass.[1,2,3,4,5,6,7,8] The impact of inadequate colostrum intake during the first hours of life on the survival and health of calves was studied in more than 2,200 animals over a five year period by the United Kingdom National Agricultural Center Calf Unit. As shown in the table below, they found that calves that received only a small amount of colostrum were six times more likely to die than those that received the required two quarts. If the animals that received a small amount of colostrum survived, they were ill almost three times as often as the calves that got enough colostrum. Getting enough high quality colostrum is essential to the health and well being of the calf and failure to do so will follow the animal for the rest of its life.

In addition to containing a high concentration of maternally derived immunoglobulins, first milking bovine colostrum is a complex resource of biologically active substances necessary to support the development and repair of cells and tissues; to assure the effective and efficient metabolism of nutrients; and to initiate and support the immune system. This is not completely surprising when we consider that it is intended for consumption by a newborn calf that

EFFECT OF COLOSTRUM INTAKE ON CALF HEALTH

Colostrum Intake	% Died	% Ill
Little	7.9	42.2
Some	3.0	24.2
Enough	1.3	15.4

has received none of the substances *in utero* that will be required for its proper development outside of the uterus and that its growth will occur at a very rapid rate, creating a huge demand for energy. The components of bovine colostrum are also compatible with almost any species and can readily convey its full benefits to other mammals, including humans, by routine dietary supplementation.

COLOSTROGENESIS–THE FORMATION OF BOVINE COLOSTRUM

The formation of colostrum in the pregnant cow is initiated about 3-4 weeks before parturition when a limited amount of fluid containing small amounts of growth factors and other transforming substances is released into the developing mammary tissue.[9,10] The process is regulated by a series of other hormones, one of the most important being progesterone, which attaches to special receptors on the cells lining the mammary gland and prevents them from secreting any fluid into the gland during most of pregnancy.[11,12] About two weeks before birth, these substances influence the appearance of specific receptors on the surface of the cells lining the mammary gland that will facilitate the transfer of materials from the mother's blood into the gland, including the immunoglobulins (antibodies) necessary to convey passive immunity to the calf after birth and various hormones and growth promoters required to induce and support development of the newborn calf.[13]

About 2 days before birth, the hormonal balance begins to shift, initiating the production of copious secretions and switching on the ability of cells in the mammary tissue to synthesize various substances, including lactose.[14,15] At birth, when the placenta is eliminated, progesterone levels fall dramatically in the mother and its inhibitory control of the secretions is removed.[12,16,17] Simultaneously, a protein-based substance develops in the cells lining the mammary gland that essentially blocks any further transfer of substances from the mother's blood into the gland.[13] The composition of the fluid in the mammary gland at birth is that of true colostrum and reflects the functional changes that have occurred in the gland up to that time; it a) has a high protein concentration, most of which is IgG; b) contains the highest concentration of growth promoters, other hormones and additional metabolically active substances; c) is low in lactose content; and d) is rich in milk fat.[18]

After birth, one of the most influential factors on the composition of subsequent secretions is physical removal of the fluid from the mammary gland. The removal of even small quantities of fluid triggers the production of copious amounts of secretion from the cells in the mammary gland.[13] Since the transfer of biologically-active substances from the mother's blood is blocked, replacement fluid will contain primarily substances synthesized by cells in the mammary gland and, thus, will be of a different composition than the fluid originally contained in the mammary gland at birth. The fluid expressed at this time is known as "transitional milk". This is further complicated by the fact that the basic composition of the colostrum changes after birth due to maternal reabsorption and does so rapidly beginning at six hours, as can be seen from the table below.[18] Thus, the highest quality bovine colostrum, containing the maximum concentration of biologically active substances, is collected in a single milking during the first six hours after parturition.

The rapidly changing composition of colostrum in the mammary gland of the mother fits together very well with events that happen in the body of the newborn calf. During the first six hours of life, the calf's stomach lining does not make any acid and there are very few, if any, enzymes present that can break down ingested proteins. Complete first milking colostrum also contains substances that inhibit the action of some enzymes. Therefore, these conditions

COMPOSITION OF LIQUID BOVINE COLOSTRUM

Hrs. After Calving	Total % Protein	Total % Fat	Total % Lactose	Total % Solids
0	17.57	5.10	2.19	26.99
6	10.00	6.85	2.71	20.46
12	6.05	3.80	3.71	14.53
24	4.52	3.40	3.98	12.77
36	3.98	3.55	3.97	12.22
48	3.74	2.80	3.97	11.46

work in favor of having the biologically active substances in complete colostrum pass through the calf's stomachs into the upper portion of the small intestine without being broken down. During the first 6-8 hours of life, an area in the upper duodenum has specialized sites where the biologically active substances can be absorbed and transported directly into the calf's bloodstream. After this period, the stomach begins to acidify, enzymes appear and the specialized absorption area in the small intestine changes dramatically so that most of the biologically active substances in colostrum are no longer absorbed. This process is aided by the fact that calves are born with a well-developed system of lymphoid tissue under their tongue and at the back of their throat that persists throughout their entire life. Many biologically active substances are absorbed through these tissues when the calf suckles its mother or a nursing bottle.[19,20,21]

THE COMPOSITION OF BOVINE COLOSTRUM

From these charts, it is very obvious how fast the relationship of the biologically active components in bovine colostrum changes after birth of the calf. Recognizing this changing relationship is extremely important in defining what bovine colostrum really is and in assuring that it contains the maximum amount of biologically active substances.[22]

COMPOSITION OF DRIED BOVINE COLOSTRUM

Hrs. After	Total % Protein	Total % Casein	Total % Albumin	Total % Fat	Total % Lactosa
0	65.10	18.82	42.02	18.90	8.11
8	48.90	17.16	30.79	33.48	13.25
12	41.64	20.65	20.37	26.15	25.53
24	35.40	21.61	11.59	26.62	31.17
30	29.42	18.78	8.80	35.95	31.33
36	32.57	22.67	8.43	29.05	32.49
48	32.64	22.95	8.64	24.43	34.64
72	32.55	22.77	8.18	26.14	36.85
96	31.73	22.62	6.92	29.60	39.83

Protein

Most of the biologically active substances in complete bovine colostrum that can convey significant health benefits are proteins. Since almost all of the beneficial proteins are conveyed from the mother's bloodstream into the colostrum before birth and the mother then begins to reabsorb them about 6-8 hours after birth, it is important to use colostrum that has been collected during a time period that will minimize the effect of the reabsorption process. Of real significance is the fact that by 24 hours after birth most of the proteins in the udder fluid can be accounted for by two individual proteins that are primarily only of nutritional value, casein and albumin.18

Fat

The milk fat in complete first milking colostrum is one the most under-rated and misunderstood components by many companies that promote bovine colostrum for human consumption. There are all kinds of stories, none of which are ever substantiated with any scientific evidence that the fat in colostrum doesn't serve any purpose and/or that having it there leads to faster deterioration of the product. Nothing could be further from the truth. In fact, one of the companies that removes the fat from what they call "colostrum" adds a component of the fat back to their dried products. They claim that this makes their "colostrum" more digestible, which was one of the functions of the fat in complete colostrum in the first place. Casein is a nutritionally valuable complete protein that is broken down in the stomach to small peptides and amino acids so that they can be absorbed and used to build new muscle protein by forming a cottage cheese-like curd in the stomach. This occurs enzymatically in the newborn and the adult and the basis for the curd that forms is the fat in the colostrum. So without it, in addition to losing some significant biologically active substances that are associated with the fat, one loses most of the nutritional value of the casein. That is part of the reason why the fat content of colostrum increases with time after birth as the amount of casein increases in the secreted fluid. Mother nature doesn't waste much and has organized the components of colostrum and their changing pattern in an efficient way to maximize the benefits to the offspring that is going to receive it.

High quality first milking bovine colostrum will contain 20-30% milk fat.[18] The milk fat in colostrum is also a very important means to deliver some of its beneficial biologically active substances.[22,23] Dissolved in or associated with the fat in colostrum are vitamins A, D, E and K; steroid hormones; corticosteroids; some growth factors; and insulin.

Lactose (milk sugar)

Approximately 10-15% of all of the solid material in high quality complete first milking colostrum will be lactose.[18] Lactose is extremely important to the calf as an immediate metabolic energy source when it is broken down to glucose and galactose by an enzyme (lactase) in the saliva and the stomach. Therefore, it makes good sense that the amount of lactose in transitional milk and mature milk increases as the calf develops rapidly during the early days of its life.

Since most people have the same enzyme (lactase) in their saliva and their digestive system, the lactose in the colostrum that they use as a dietary supplement can provide the same ready source of metabolic energy. However, there are "lactose intolerant" individuals who have problems digesting lactose because their body produces too little or none of the lactase enzyme. The amount of lactose in first milking colostrum collected within 6 hours after birth is about one-half of what it is at 12 hours after birth and one-third of what it becomes by 24 hours. Therefore, high quality complete first milking colostrum collected within 6 hours after birth can be used as a dietary supplement by more people without potentially having them suffer the discomforts associated with lactose intolerance.

OTHER COMPOSITIONAL CONSIDERATIONS

The following comparative facts about colostrum and milk further stress the value of a complete first milking colostrum in maximizing the health related benefits.[22]

- Colostrum contains 10 times more vitamin A than milk.
- Colostrum contains 3 times more vitamin D than milk.
- Colostrum contains at least 10 times more iron than milk.
- Colostrum contains more calcium, phosphorous and magnesium than milk.

BIOLOGICALLY ACTIVE COMPONENTS

The biologically active components in complete first milking colostrum can be divided into categories based upon the health aspect where they exert their greatest influence. In some cases the functions of these components can be clearly separated into such categories, while, in many cases, the dividing line is clouded. The major categories are the Immune Factors, the Growth Factors and the Metabolic Factors. It is very important to recognize that most of the very broad claims made by many suppliers of colostrum for human consumption about what these substances do are based upon very specialized studies in experimental animals and represent the company's interpretation of the results and not necessarily that of the original scientific investigator.

IMMUNE FACTORS

To comprehend what the Immune Factors are in high quality first milking colostrum and what they do, it is important to recognize that some of these components have one or more effects on the overall regulation and functioning of the immune system (immuno-regulating substances), while others are very restricted in what they can do and their benefits are usually very localized in the body, ordinarily exerting their effects primarily in the gut (gut protective substances).

Immuno-regulating substances

Thymosin (alpha & beta chains). A hormone composed of two protein-based chains that are separately present in bovine colostrum. The chains act on the thymus gland independently or in concert with each other to stimulate activation, development and maintenance of the immune system.[24,25,26]

Proline-rich peptide (PRP), a/k/a thymulin. A hormone-like small protein that acts upon the thymus and other organs associated with the immune system to keep them from over-reacting to an insult.[27]

Cytokines. Small proteins produced by various cells in the body that induce the generation of specialized types of white blood cells, signal them to come to the site of an insult and help in their passage through tissues.[27,28]

Lymphokines. Proteins of varying sizes that are produced by different types of white blood cells that tell related cells to transform themselves into more functional cell types that can release substances capable of destroying an invading microorganism.[29,30]

Immunoglobulins (IgG, IgM, IgA). Complex proteins, better known as antibodies, that make up a significant portion of the proteins found in complete first milking colostrum. These antibodies were produced by the mother's immune system in response to her exposure to many different microorganisms during her lifetime and then transferred into the colostrum prior to birth of the calf. There is no evidence that any of these antibodies are found intact in the blood of individuals who ingest colostrum by mouth. However, many of these antibodies are reactive against bacteria, viruses and fungi that infect the gastrointestinal tract of humans and there is scientific evidence that some of them can survive passage through the digestive system.[31,32]

Transfer factors. Small proteins produced in response to the body's exposure to certain types of microorganisms, particularly those that reside in deep tissues for a long period of time, like *Mycobacterium tuberculosis*. They are specific for a particular microorganism and are carried inside of certain types of specialized white blood cells. Transfer factors have limited effectiveness alone in defending the body against infection by such microorganisms, but, rather, act in concert with various white blood cells and other factors in an attempt to keep the microorganisms under control. [33,34,35]

Lactoferrin. A mineral-binding carrier protein that attaches to available iron. Certain aerobic bacteria, like *E. coli*, require iron to reproduce and, therefore, lactoferrin is an effective substance, when operating in the presence of a specific antibody, to impede the growth of some microorganisms in the gut. A broad number of additional claims have been made by some providers of colostrum for human consumption regarding the application of lactoferrin as an immuno-regulating substance with antiviral, antibacterial and anti-tumor properties. To date, none of these claims have been adequately substantiated through properly controlled studies. [36,37]

Transferrin. Another mineral-binding carrier protein that attaches to available iron and can act independently or in concert with lactoferrin to impede the growth of certain aerobic bacteria, particularly in the gut. [36]

Lysozyme. A very powerful enzyme that is capable of attaching itself to the cell wall of certain pathogenic bacteria and degrading selected proteins, leaving holes in the wall of the bacteria. [38]

Lactoperoxidase. A mildly effective enzyme that can also attach to the wall of certain bacteria, degrade other selected proteins and interfere with the ability of the bacteria to replicate. [38]

Xanthine Oxidase. Another mildly effective enzyme that can also attach to the wall of certain bacteria, degrade different proteins than those affected by lactoperoxidase and also interfere with the ability of the bacteria to replicate. [38]

White blood cells (leukocytes). Primarily three types of functional white blood cells are present in colostrum, including neutrophils, macrophages and polymorphonuclear cells. Each has the ability to phagocytize microorganisms and other foreign bodies and apply substances carried internally to the destruction of the microorganisms. Their functions are dramatically enhanced when antibodies first attach to the microorganisms. [22]

Oligosaccharides and glycoconjugates. Complex carbohydrates (sugars) that can adhere to specific sites on the inner surface of the gastrointestinal tract and prevent the attachment of microorganisms. [39]

GROWTH FACTORS

Growth hormone. Very small quantities of growth hormone are found in complete first milking colostrum, but that is all that is required since this hormone is extremely potent. It has a direct effect on almost every cell type and significantly influences the proliferation of new cells, particularly their rate of generation. Scientific studies have shown that continued ingestion of small amounts of growth hormone are beneficial in limiting the ongoing deterioration of cells associated with the aging process. [40,41]

Insulin-like growth factors (IGFs). Insulin-like growth factor-1 (IGF-1) and its closely related counterpart insulin-like growth factor-2 (IGF-2) are potent hormones that are found in association with almost all cells in the body. They are part of a group of more than 90 different proteins, called the "IGF Binding Protein (IGFBP) Superfamily", that is responsible for the processes by which cells grow and reproduce. These substances are also responsible for maintenance of the metabolic pathways by which cells convert glucose to glycogen, a primary metabolic energy resource, and assemble amino acids to create proteins. The key event that triggers the functions of the various proteins in the IGFBP Superfamily is the attachment of IGF-1 to a specific receptor site on the surface of a cell. Many of the growth factors found in colostrum and previously defined by their functions are now considered part of the IGFBP Superfamily. This includes the following substances, among others. [42,43]

Transforming growth factors A & B. Induces the transformation of cells from an immature form to a mature, functional status.

Epithelial growth factor. Involved in the generation and maintenance of cells in the epithelial layers of the skin.

Fibroblast growth factor. Associated with the regeneration of various types of tissue, including skin and other organs.

Platelet-derived growth factor. Responsible for the generation of cells and functions associated with blood clotting.

METABOLIC FACTORS

Leptin. A small hormone-like protein that can suppress appetite, enhance metabolic rate and lead to body weight reduction. Mature fat cells (adipocytes) release leptin in the presence of insulin, which is also found in colostrum. Insulin-producing pancreatic beta-cells have receptor sites for leptin and it is believed that the size of fat cells may be a major factor in determining the amount of leptin released. The binding of leptin to its receptors in the presence of insulin initiates a cascade of chemical signals to the hypothalamus resulting in appetite suppression and the triggering of fat metabolism in the liver. Leptin deficiency may be associated with obesity, particularly in diabetic individuals. [44,45,46]

Insulin. A hormone required for the effective metabolic utilization of glucose. Insulin binds to specific receptor sites on cells, facilitating their interaction with IGF-1 and, thus, initiating the conversion of glucose to glycogen, a major source of metabolic energy.

Vitamin-binding proteins. Smaller proteins that act as carriers to deliver B-complex vitamins to the body. Carrier proteins and the associated vitamins folate (B6), B12 and orotic acid are found in colostrum.

Fat-associated vitamins. Significant quantities of vitamins A, D, E and K are dissolved in or associated with the fat in colostrum.

Mineral-binding proteins. In addition to interfering with the replication of certain microorganisms, the iron-binding proteins, lactoferrin and transferrin, also serve to capture iron from ingested sources and present it in a form that can be readily absorbed by the body. Lactoferrin can also bind copper and deliver it in a form suitable for absorption by the body. In addition, there are two carrier proteins in colostrum that assist in the absorption of calcium. They are casein, which is also an abundant source of amino acids to build new protein molecules, and alpha-lactalbumin, which is present in colostrum very soon after birth.

Cyclic adenosine monophosphate (cAMP). A phosphorylated nucleotide in a high-energy state that is applicable to energy transfer in metabolism. This is the lowest energy form of adenosine triphosphate (ATP), the primary energy transfer molecule in normal metabolism. AMP can be recycled to ATP through existent intracellular pathways and, thus, colostrum can serve as a resource for these energy transfer substances.

Enzyme inhibitors. These have been called "permeability factors" by other manufacturers, but are actually small proteins that slow down or inhibit the breakdown of proteins by certain enzymes. They provide limited protection to the immune, growth and metabolic factors as they pass through the digestive tract.

Health-related benefits of colostrum ingestion

High quality first milking bovine colostrum is not a panacea that will cure every disease as claimed by many distributors of colostrum products. However, bovine colostrum is an amazing resource of substances necessary to support the development and repair of cells and tissues, assure the effective and efficient metabolism of nutrients and establish and maintain a healthy immune system. As such, it represents a very dynamic means to stabilize bodily functions that are frequently out of control in various disease states. In other circumstances, these bodily functions may just need the boost that colostrum can provide to ward off disease.

The use of colostrum for its health-related benefits is not a new concept. In India, where cows are sacred, colostrum is delivered to the home with the milk and is used for medicinal purposes to treat everything from age-related symptoms to the common cold. This practice began several thousand years ago with Ayurvedic physicians and sacred healers known as Rishis. In the Scandinavian countries, the birth of a calf is celebrated by the making of a pudding for human consumption from the extra colostrum after the calf is fed. This practice has gone on for centuries and is intended to promote good health. Research conducted in these countries as early as the late 18th century showed the benefits of colostrum on the health and development of cattle and laid the groundwork for the early medicinal use of colostrum by humans. The early Amish farmers in America practiced this same ritual.

GASTROINTESTINAL DISEASES

Leaky gut syndrome is a very common condition wherein the mucosal lining of the small intestine becomes very inflamed and unusually large spaces develop between the cells that make up the mucosal lining. The large spaces between the cells allows bacteria, viruses, fungi and other potentially toxic material to enter the bloodstream and other parts of the body. In addition, undigested proteins, carbohydrates and fats can pass through the intestinal lining and can represent a serious health risk.

Medical research has shown that the inflammatory process responsible for leaky gut syndrome can be initiated in many different ways, including the following.

- Excess ingestion of alcohol and/or drinks containing caffeine.
- Continuous use of antibiotics resulting in destruction of the inherent bacterial flora in the intestine.
- Ingestion of foods contaminated by certain bacteria or parasites.
- Routine ingestion of corticosteroids, such as prednisone, and/or non-steroidal anti-inflammatory drugs like aspirin or ibuprofen.
- Consumption of large quantities of highly refined carbohydrates, such as the sugar found in candy, cookies, cakes and soft drinks.

Routine dietary supplementation with high quality bovine colostrum can be of substantial value when this condition occurs.[47,48] In leaky gut syndrome, the individual's normal protective mechanisms against invading infectious bacteria, viruses, fungi and parasites are severely compromised. Colostrum contains a diversity of antibodies that can bind to invading microorganisms and hold them in check while they are engulfed and destroyed by white blood cells arriving in the area. The most important of these antibody molecules in colostrum are of the IgA class. They not only attach themselves to an invading microorganism, but are also able to stick to tissues, holding the pathogen in a fixed position and making it more susceptible to destruction by white blood cells. The lactoferrin transferrin, and enzymes in colostrum also significantly aid the entire process of destroying invading microorganisms.

The growth factors in colostrum, growth hormone (GH) and the insulin-like growth factors (IGFs), are also of substantial benefit. It is well documented in the scientific literature that the influence of growth hormone on the proliferation of new cells in the body operates primarily through what is known as the GH/IGF axis where the presence of growth hormone enhances the many effects of the insulin-like growth factors. [49] IGF-1 is like the captain of a ship. It directs the many activities of a multitude of specialized proteins found in every cell in the body, including the process by which the cell grows and reproduces itself. IGF-1 is also responsible for maintenance of the metabolic pathways by which the cell uses glucose to make energy and builds proteins from amino acids. Therefore, the presence of sufficient quantities of growth hormone and the insulin-like growth factors in the circulation will support the repair of damaged tissue. [50,51]

Leaky gut syndrome also results in significant mineral deficiencies due to damage to the carrier proteins by the associated inflammatory process. Many essential minerals are not absorbed into the body unless they are attached to specialized carrier proteins. Two of the most important minerals, iron and copper, bind to the lactoferrin and transferrin found in colostrum, which function as effective carrier proteins. In addition, the casein in colostrum, which is an excellent source of the essential amino acids that the body cannot make, is also a highly functional carrier protein for calcium, allowing it to be effectively absorbed from the small intestine.

Individuals afflicted with ulcerative colitis or Crohn's disease also usually benefit significantly from routine dietary supplementation with high quality bovine colostrum. [52,53] First, dairy cows are usually exposed during their lifetime to pathogenic forms of both *E. coli* and *Mycobacterium paratuberculosis,* infectious agents presumed to be associated with these conditions. Thus, the colostrum from these animals will contain immunoglobulins directed against both of these organisms. In addition, as for leaky gut syndrome, the broad diversity of antibodies against a multitude of potentially pathogenic microorganisms present in high quality colostrum will also be beneficial. Further, as also discussed above, the presence of sufficient quantities of growth hormone and the insulin-like growth factors found in bovine colostrum will support the repair of damaged tissue.

Enteric infections with potentially pathogenic bacteria, including coliforms, like *E. coli, Staphylococcus* species, *Streptococcus* species, and *Salmonella* species can also be abated. Antibodies to all of these pathogens are found in high quality colostrum. [54,55,56] However, the antibodies are most beneficial when they are present early in an infection and, therefore, maximum protection is afforded against enteric infections by routine ingestion of high quality colostrum as a dietary supplement. In addition, as in leaky bowel syndrome, the lactoferrin, transferrin and enzymes present in colostrum will aid in destroying an invading pathogen once the antibody molecules immobilize it.

Controlled studies in humans have shown that substances present in bovine colostrum inhibit the binding of *Helicobactor pylori*, the causative agent in ulcer lesions, to receptors on the intestinal wall. [57,58]

RESPIRATORY HEALTH

In dealing with something as elusive as the common cold or as invasive as influenza, the best offense is a good defense. Coupling a nutritious diet with a program of exercise and routine supplementation with high quality bovine colostrum is the best possible defense. As we age, our immune system loses its ability to regulate itself and to respond to a challenge efficiently. This occurs primarily because the thymus, a glandular structure in the upper chest that is considered the seat of the immune system, begins to shrink after puberty and almost disappears by the time we are 50-60 years old. [59,60,61] T-lymphocytes (T-cells) are generated from stem cells in the bone marrow and mature in the thymus. Some of these cells, called Killer T-lymphocytes, generate cell-mediated responses and directly destroy abnormal cells that have specific sites on their surface that are recognized by the Killer T- lymphocytes. Helper/Suppressor T-lymphocytes, a second type of cell, regulate the immune system by controlling the strength and quality of every immune response. It has been shown that the thymus can be restored to normal function by the growth factors in colostrum. [62,63,64,65,66] In addition, colostrum contains specific hormones that regulate the functions of the thymus and other substances that help to keep the immune system under control and poised to respond to possible infections before they become established. [67]

CARDIOVASCULAR HEALTH

High quality first milking bovine colostrum does not contain any cholesterol and can be used safely by individuals with high serum cholesterol and high triglycerides. In fact, there are biologically active substances present in bovine colostrum that would be very beneficial to individuals at risk for atherosclerotic plaque formation. Bovine colostrum contains leptin, a hormone-like substance that not only suppresses appetite, but also orchestrates how the body uses and incorporates fat.

Growth hormone has been shown to work in concert with IGF-1 in the functioning and repair of heart muscle.[68] Receptors for both growth hormone and IGF-1 are found on all heart muscle cells and scientific evidence indicates that growth hormone may act directly on the heart, whereas the effects of IGF-1 may be indirect and operate through separate hormonal pathways.[69,70] Research studies have also shown that both growth hormone and IGF-1 have stimulatory effects on heart muscle cells and it is believed that this occurs through the pathway by which the cells use calcium.[71] It has also been shown that administration of growth hormone to patients with congestive heart failure can induce a marked improvement in heart function and clinical status.[72]

METABOLIC HEALTH

Both Type I and II diabetes have an associated genetic component through which individuals appear to be predisposed. Diabetics also have low levels of IGF-1 in their circulation.[49,73] Daily supplementation of the diet of the diabetic patient with a high quality first milking bovine colostrum will provide a functional source for the restoration of diminished levels of IGF-1, resulting in increased utilization of available glucose. This becomes extremely important for the Type I diabetic to assure effective and controlled utilization of available glucose once his/her insulin levels are restored. In the Type II diabetic, where sufficient insulin is available, it has been shown experimentally that restoration of reduced IGF-1 levels results in an enhancement of glucose utilization with a corresponding diminution of glucose levels in the blood and urine.[74]

AUTOIMMUNE HEALTH

Diseases such as systemic lupus erythematosus (SLE) and rheumatoid arthritis, among others, are complex clinical conditions with variable outcomes. All of the these diseases represent an immune system that is out of control and could be restored and regulated through routine dietary supplementation with a high quality first milking colostrum. As indicated above (see Respiratory Diseases), as we age, our immune system loses its ability to regulate itself efficiently, primarily because the thymus begins to shrink after puberty and essentially disappears by the time we are 50-60 years old. Scientific studies have shown that the thymus can be restored to normal function by IGF-1[62,63,64,65,66], the levels of which diminish in the circulation with age. In addition, colostrum contains a) specific hormones, the alpha and beta chains of thymosin, that are known to regulate the functions of the thymus; and b) proline-rich peptide (PRP), a/k/a thymulin, that has been shown to keep the immune system under control.[35,36,37,67]

It is also well documented that IGF-1 and the associated Superfamily of proteins found in colostrum operate in concert with growth hormone in the regeneration and repair of damaged cells.[75] Routine dietary supplementation with high quality bovine colostrum is, therefore, desirable for individuals afflicted with autoimmune diseases in order to assure that sufficient levels of IGF-1 and growth hormone are continuously available in the circulation. In addition, since IGF-1 is responsible for directing the conversion of glucose to glycogen and glycogen is a primary metabolic energy resource, such dietary supplementation could also help such individuals overcome the associated lethargy normally experienced with such diseases.

ACQUIRED IMMUNE DEFICIENCY SYNDROME (AIDS)

The primary site for maturation of T-lymphocytes and their release into the body in response to an insult is the thymus gland. Unfortunately, as we age this organ shrinks and loses its functions and valuable immune response capabilities are diminished or lost. This is a serious consideration in the individual infected with the human immunodeficiency virus (HIV), since the immune system is the primary focus of attack by the virus. As indicated above, the IGF-1 found in colostrum has been shown to be capable of restoring the thymus to its normal functioning capacity. In addition, colostrum contains both the alpha and beta chains of thymosin, which are hormones that have been shown to operate independently and in concert to promote the functions of the thymus. Separate studies in experimental animals have also shown that daily ingestion of a high quality bovine colostrum results in a more expedient and effective response by the immune system when a potentially infectious microorganism challenges the body. In dealing with infectious diseases like AIDS, experts agree that the best offense is a good defense and that having the healthiest possible immune system, that is more capable of responding to a challenge, will likely assist in warding off infection and/or help in prolonging the development of the disease.

Other substances found in bovine colostrum may also prove beneficial to AIDS patients. In limited studies, lactoferrin, an iron-binding component of colostrum, has been shown to completely prevent infection with certain viruses to which the AIDS patient may become susceptible.[36,76,77] Independent scientific studies have also shown that the lactoferrin found in bovine colostrum is at least twice as potent as that found naturally in humans.[37]

The antibodies present in high quality bovine colostrum have also proven to be effective in helping to limit the severe diarrhea usually associated with the opportunistic enteric infections experienced by many AIDS patients. Actual studies conducted in persons suffering severe diarrhea in association with immune system deficiency evidenced that over half of the patients treated with bovine colostrum remained free of diarrhea for at least four weeks. [78,79]

The wasting associated with the evolution of the disease in AIDS patients represents the destruction of muscle mass and is usually paralleled by the development of extreme fatigue and loss of energy. As described above, having a sufficient quantity of IGF-1 in the circulation, as would occur by routine dietary supplementation with high quality colostrum, assures the effective and efficient conversion of glucose to glycogen, supporting metabolic energy requirements to help overcome the developing lethargy and fatigue. In addition, having sufficient IGF-1 available also helps to assure proper utilization of amino acids in the building of proteins required to maintain muscle mass.

BODY COMPOSITION AND PERFORMANCE

Supplementation with bovine colostrum has been shown to affect body composition in a study using a small group of trained athletes. After 8 weeks of daily supplementation with 20 grams of a powdered colostrum preparation, lean body mass increased significantly in the colostrum group compared to a placebo group given whey. There was no improvement in exercise performance in either group. [80] Other workers found increased levels of serum insulin, IGF-1 and immunoglobulins in a group of athletes consuming a liquid colostrum drink daily for 8 training days, with no improvement in vertical jump ability. [81]

Other studies have found that supplementation with a "concentrated bovine colostrum protein powder" daily for 8 weeks did not increase serum IGF-1 levels, but appeared to improve recovery from a run to exhaustion test during the second half of the 8 week period. The placebo used was whey. [82] A second study by the same research group using the same colostrum preparation and dosage and a whey placebo found that performance by trained young women rowers in the colostrum group improved by the ninth week of a 9 week training program, as compared to placebo. [83] In a separate study, routine daily supplementation with a colostrum powder was shown to increase the physical stamina of field hockey players. [84]

In other studies, resistance-trained subjects received either bovine colostrum, a casein-whey placebo, colostrum + an additional supplement (containing creatine, carnitine, and taurine), or the supplement only, for 12 weeks. All subjects consumed the same amount of protein. The colostrum + supplement group showed a 5.7 lb increase in fat free mass (FFM), compared to 2.8 lbs in the colostrum group and 4.2 lbs in the supplement only group.[85] Measurements of training adaptations indicated that the colostrum + supplement group had the greatest improvements in bench press and leg press performance.[86]

SAFETY

There appear to be no adverse effects due to the use of colostrum as a dietary supplement. However, the presence of IGF in colostrum and the reported increase in serum IGF levels following colostrum use has raised some concerns about its safety. Multiple studies have shown that there is an elevated level of IGF-1 in the circulation of patients with certain types of malignancies including, prostate cancer[87,88], breast cancer[89,90], colorectal cancer[91] and acute lymphoblastic leukemia[92]. The fact that IGF-1 is a growth promoting substance led to the erroneous conclusion by some that it is a causative agent in malignant disease that would promote the growth of tumors. However, more recent studies have shown that tumor cells have poorly functioning or modified receptors for IGF-1 on their surface, and, since the binding of IGF-1 to a cell surface receptor triggers many functions in all cells, unbound, available IGF-1 will back-up in the circulation.[93,94,95,96] Therefore, the higher levels of IGF-1 found in the circulation of cancer patients are a manifestation of their tumor and not a causative factor. A similar manifestation of receptor impairment and commensurate alteration in circulating levels of IGF-1 is seen in diabetic individuals.[97]

COLLECTION AND PROCESSING OF COLOSTRUM

The antibodies found in the blood of a pregnant cow that are eventually transferred into the colostrum were all derived by the immune system of that cow in response to foreign substances to which the cow had been exposed during its lifetime. These foreign substances include the various vaccines administered to protect the animal against different potential disease-causing microorganisms; clinical and non-clinical contagious infections experienced as a result of contact with other members of the herd, including microorganisms present in their excrement; and microorganisms vectored from handling and contact with equipment and other species.

Some distributors of colostrum state that colostrum should only come from cows that are pasture-fed since that provides more antibody diversity. Although it is theoretically possible that some pathogens may be present in the soil and be vectored to the cow, this is highly unlikely since microorganisms that would ordinarily be found in clean soil and on grasses suitable for grazing would not be pathogenic to mammals—otherwise all of the animals in the herd would be sick most of the time. Pathogens found in a pasture or any other environment would most likely be present as a result of animal excrement.

In the United States, it was recognized many years ago that open pasturing of dairy cows, including breeding and unsupported calf delivery in the pasture environment, was not conducive to good herd management practices and led to a higher incidence of disease; affected milk production volumes and the quality of milk. It also failed to provide the support necessary to assure that calves received adequate volumes of colostrum of sufficient quality to promote their proper development. A large number of dairy farms in the United States have shifted to a dual technique that allows the cows both lot and pasture. The animals are kept either inside of a structure or outside within clean, fenced environments and fed a well-defined diet containing the required nutrients to assure effective development and maintenance of their health status. These areas can be cleaned routinely, either manually or automatically, to assure removal of excrement. The animals in such environments are frequently divided into groups reflecting the number of lactation cycles they have experienced and their average milk production capabilities. This approach allows the dairy producer to more effectively control disease development and to recognize and separate animals with problems, regulate milking schedules, and control the quality and flavor of the milk.

It has also become a dairy industry standard in the United States that all pregnant cows due to deliver are monitored every 1-2 hours around the clock. For this purpose, most dairy farms have a "maternity ward" away from the main herd that allows for the required monitoring and facilitates calf handling and colostrum collection within the first six hours after birth. It is also very common for producers to prevent newborn calves from suckling as they receive better care and better colostrum delivery if they are nursed by hand. In addition, when calves are removed from their mothers at birth, they have less exposure to the maternity area, decreasing disease transmission through contact with fecal material and the mother's teats.

Companies marketing the highest quality bovine colostrum usually have access to at least 500 dairy herds averaging about 300 cows each. Since cows are biological creatures and, thus, will not all have the same levels of biologically active components in their individual colostrum, collecting from a large number of animals in different herds and manufacturing from large pools of colostrum supports the control of product uniformity and assures a maximum level of all of the beneficial components in each production lot.

COLLECTION AND PROCESSING

True colostrum must be obtained in the first milking taken during the 6 hours after birth of the calf. Many years ago the United States Department of Health defined colostrum as the "milk" collected in the first six milkings after birth. This was done to keep colostrum out of milk intended for human consumption since it was believed then that it was only suitable for consumption by the calf. However, science has now significantly advanced our understanding of what colostrum really is, how it is formed and the many benefits that it can convey to humans as well as calves. We now know that, in the pregnant cow, colostrum formation ceases at birth and that the mother begins to reabsorb the active components about 6-8 hours after birth if the colostrum is not collected. We also know that the colostrum should be collected in one unit since, as soon as a small volume of colostrum is removed, a much larger volume of transitional milk will enter the udder and dilute the residual colostrum.

Apparently, the scientific facts have not reached every manufacturer of colostrum since some of them still market "colostrum" that is collected from multiple milkings after the birth of the calf. This obviously results in much more "product" per cow, but the resulting colostrum powders are deficient in many of the most beneficial components and the remaining constituents have been significantly diluted. Thus, they will never provide the same range of benefits that can be realized with high quality first milking colostrum.

High quality colostrum must be collected under very stringent conditions. These conditions require that a) colostrum be included only from cows that have experienced three or more live births to maximize the quality of bioactives and assure antibody diversity; b) no colostrum be collected from any animal evidencing any form of inflammation of the udder; and c) no colostrum evidencing blood, mucus, somatic cell clumps or strings, other foreign matter or discoloration be included.

Colostrum should be frozen immediately after it is collected and then transferred as quickly as possible, in the frozen state, to the processing facility. This is very important since no milk product is completely free of bacteria when it is collected and leaving the colostrum in the liquid state would encourage some bacteria to reproduce, spoiling the colostrum and, perhaps, generating large numbers of disease-causing bacteria.

Some colostrum manufacturers claim that freezing will destroy the biologically active components and make them insoluble and impossible to absorb in the body. Freezing, in itself, does not alter the water-soluble nature of organic substances such as those found in colostrum. For this to occur in colostrum would require that the configuration of the many protein molecules be changed, such as occurs when they are heat-denatured at excessive temperatures, often causing them to precipitate from solution. In fact, freezing of protein solutions is the principal means of storage by laboratories to maintain the integrity and biological activity of molecules. It is well established in scientific practice that the method used for thawing frozen specimens, rather than freezing, can denature proteins and, to avoid this, the protein solution must be thawed slowly at a temperature that does not exceed 98.6° F/37° C.

When the individual colostrum units arrive at the processing facility, they must be thawed very gently and then examined and tested thoroughly to assure their quality. They can then be pooled together and processed by specialized methods that maintain the integrity of all of the biologically-active components to a) destroy bacteria that may have been present; and b) remove at least 98% of the water to yield a dry powder with good storage capabilities. These are complex and costly procedures and if a manufacturer cannot provide assurances that they have been carefully followed, it is highly likely that the resulting "colostrum" powder will yield few, if any, benefits no matter when or how it was collected.

COMPLETE COLOSTRUM

To maximize the benefits from a colostrum powder, it must not only meet the above criteria, but it must also be derived from complete colostrum that is unadulterated and contains everything found in true colostrum as it is generated in the cow. In addition, it should contain only complete colostrum and no additives or supplements that might change the characteristics of the biologically active components or interfere with their effectiveness.

Some companies that market so-called "colostrum" physically or chemically remove some of the components, like the fat, claiming that it avoids the development of rancidity and increases the shelf-life of the powder. This approach not only changes the composition of the colostrum and the relationship of the active components, but also removes some very valuable constituents, like the fat-soluble vitamins and a portion of the growth factors. The argument that removing the fat increases the shelf life is, in itself, completely without scientific merit since rancidity in dairy products is associated with fluid materials and is not a consideration for a properly dried colostrum powder.

In addition to acting as a carrier vehicle for certain components, the fat in colostrum plays a very significant role in assuring that the maximum benefits are available from ingested colostrum powder. High quality colostrum also contains a significant amount of casein, a complex, complete protein that contains beneficial essential amino acids. When complete colostrum enters the stomach, an enzyme (rennin) naturally present there acts upon the casein and fat to form a soft cottage cheese-like curd that entrains the active components and protects them from exposure to stomach acid and digestive enzymes. This helps to assure that as much of each biologically active component as possible reaches the small intestine, where absorption into the blood stream occurs.

CONCLUSIONS

Colostrum reflects the evolutionary development of a unique composition that will serve the needs of the offspring for which it is intended. The most unique of the colostrums from mammalian species occurs in bovine species where everything required for the development of a healthy, productive offspring is provided in the colostrum. As such, it provides a specialized resource that offers the broadest possible spectrum of biologically active substances that can promote the development of a sound body mass, assure effective and efficient metabolism and support the activation and maintenance of a fully functional immune system capable of combating potential insults from microorganisms and other deleterious sources. Bovine colostrum is also compatible with almost any species and can readily convey its full benefits to humans by routine dietary supplementation without any significant adverse effects.

However, it is very important to recognize that all colostrum products are not the same and, despite the claims made by their manufacturers, they do not all contain every beneficial component at an optimum concentration and, in many cases, they have been manipulated and may be missing some of the essential components. When choosing a colostrum product, one should be certain that it is made from only first milking bovine colostrum collected within 6 hours after birth of the calf and that the colostrum is "complete" and that none of the components have been removed, including the fat.

REFERENCES

1   Blum JW, Baumrucker CR; Colostral and milk insulin-like growth factors and related substances: mammary gland and neonatal (intestinal and systemic) targets, Domest Anim Endocrinol 2002; 23(1-2):101-10.

2   Buhler C, Hammon R; Small intestinal morphology in eight day old calves fed colostrum for different durations or only milk replacer and treated with insulin-like growth factor and growth hormone, J Anim Sci 1998; 76(3):758-65.

3   Hammon HM, Blum JW; Feeding different amounts of colostrum or only milk replacer modifies receptors of intestinal insulin-like growth factors and insulin in calves, Domest Anim Endocrinol 2002; 22(3):155-68.

4   Nocek JE, et al; Influence of neonatal colostrum administration, immunoglobulin, and continued feeding of colostrum on calf gain, health and serum protein, J Dairy Sci 1984; 67(2):319-33.

5   Nussbaum A, et al; Growth performance and metabolic and endocrine traits in calves pair-fed by bucket or by automate starting in the neonatal period, J Anim Sci 2002; 80(6):1545-55.

6   Korhonen H, et al; Bovine milk antibodies for health, Brit J Nutr 2000; 84(Suppl1):S135-46.

7   McGuire TC, et al; Failure of colostral immunoglobulin transfer in calves dying from infectious disease, J Am Vet Med Assoc 1976; 169:713-8.

8   Quigley JD, et al; Formulation of colostrum supplements, colostrum replacers and acquisition of passive immunity in neonatal calves, J Dairy Sci 2001; 84:2059-65.

9   Plaut K; Role of epidermal growth factor and transforming growth factors in mammary development and lactation, J Dairy Sci 1993; 76(6):1526-38.

10 Plath A, at al; Expression of transforming growth factors alpha and beta-1 messenger RNA in the bovine mammary gland during different stages of development and lactation, J Endocrinol 1997; 155(3):501-11.

11 Delouis C; Physiology of colostrum production, Ann Vet Res 1978; 9(2):193-203.

12 Forsyth IA; The Endocrinology of Lactation, T.B. Mepham, ed.; Elsevier Science Publishers 1983; pp 309-49.

13 Barrington GM, et al; Regulation of immunoglobulin G1 receptor: effect of prolactin on in vivo expression of the bovine mammary gland receptor, J Endocrinol 1999; 163(1):25-31.

14 Akers RM; Lactogenic hormones: binding sites, mammary growth, secretory cell differentiation and milk biosynthesis in ruminants, J Dairy Sci 1985; 68(2):501-19.

15 Barrington GM, et al; Regulation of colostrogenesis in cattle, Livest Prod Sci 2000; 70(1-2):95-104.

16 Guy MA, et al; Regulation of colostrum formation in beef and dairy cows, J Dairy Sci 1994; 77(10):3002-7.

17 Tucker HA, Lactation and its Hormonal Control, in The Physiology of Reproduction, 2nd edition, E. Knobil & J. Neill eds.; Raven Press Ltd. 1994; pp 1065-110.

18 Fundamentals of Dairy Chemistry, 2nd Ed, B.H. Webb, A.H. Johnson, J.A. Alford eds; The AVI Publishing Co., Westport, CT, 1978.

19 Quigley JD, Kost CJ, Wolfe TM; Absorption of protein and IgG in calves fed a colostrum supplement or replacer, J Dairy Sci 2002; 85(5): 1243-8.

20 Schams D; Einspanier R; Growth hormone, IGF-1 and insulin in mammary gland secretions before and after parturition and possibility of their transfer into a calf, Endocrine Regulation 1991; 25(1-2): 139-143.

21 Xu R; Development of newborn GI tract and its relationship to colostrum/milk intake: a review, Reprod Fertil Devel 1996; 8(11):35-48.

22 Hurley WL; Animal Science 308 (on-line): The Neonate and Colostrum, University of Illinois Urbana-Champagne; 2000, 11 pgs. {http//:classes.aces.uiuc.edu/AnSci308].

23 Kuhn NJ; The Biochemistry of Lactogenesis. In Biochemistry of Lactation, T.B. Mepham, ed.; Elseviers Science Publishers 1983; pp 309-49.

24 Ancell CD, et al; Thymosin alpha-1, Am J Health Syst Pharm 2001; 58(10):879-85.

25 Li QY, et al; Thymosin beta-4 regulation, expression and function in aortic valve interstitial cells, J Heart Valve Dis 2002; 11(5):726-35.

26 Yarmola M, et al; Formation and implications of ternary complex of profiling, thymosin beta-4, and actin, J Biol Chem 2001; 276(49):455-63.

27 Kanaan SA, et al; Thymulin reduces the hyperalgesia and cytokine upregulation induced by leishmaniasis in mice, Brain Behav Immunol 2002; 16(4):450-60.

28 Solomons NW; Modulation of the immune system and the response against pathogens with bovine colostrum concentrates, Eur J Clin Nutr 2002; 56(S3):S24-8.

29 Pido-Lopez J, et al; Molecular quantitation of thymic output in mice and the effect of IL-7, Eur J Immunol 2002; 32(10):2827-36.

30 Saito H, et al; Topical antigen provocation increases the number of immunoreactive IL-4, IL-5 and IL-6 positive cells in the nasal mucosa of patients with perennial allergic rhinitis, Int Arch Allergy Immunol 1997; 114(1):81-5.

31 Nord J, et al; Treatment with bovine hyperimmune colostrum of crypto-sporidial diarrhea in AIDS patients, AIDS 1990; 4(6):581-4.

32 Rump JA, et al; Treatment of diarrhea in human immunodeficiency virus-infected patients with immunoglobulins from bovine colostrum, Clin Investig 1992; 70(7):588-94.

33 Kirkpatrick, CH; Activities and characteristics of transfer factors; Biotherapy 1996; 9(1-3): 13-16.

34 Kirkpatrick, CH; Transfer factors: identification of conserved sequences in transfer factor molecules; Mol. Med. 2000 Apr.; 6(4): 332-41.

35 Lawrence, HS, Borkowsky, W; Transfer factor - current status and future prospects; Biotherapy 1996; 9(1-3):1-5.

36   Lonnerdal B, Iyer S; Lactoferrin: molecular structure and biological function, Ann Rev Nutrition 1995; 13:93-110.

37   Brock J; Lactoferrin: a multifunctional immunoregulatory protein. Immunol Today 1995; 16(9):417-19.

38   Kussendrager KD, van Hooijdonk AC; Lactoperoxidase: physico-chemical properties, occurrence, mechanism of action and applications, Brit J Nutr 2000; 84 (Suppl 1): S19-25.

39   Gopal PK, Gill HS; Oligosaccharides and glycoconjugates in bovine milk and colostrum, Brit J Nutr 2000; 84(Suppl 1):S69-74.

40   Cameron CM, et al; The acute effects of growth hormone on amino acid transport and protein synthesis are due to its insulin-like action, Endocrinol 1988; 122(2):471-4.

41   Shing Y, Elagabrun M; Purification and characteristics of a bovine colostrum-derived growth factor, Molec Endocrinol 1987; 25(3):335-40.

42   Hwa V, et al; The insulin-like growth factor binding protein (IGFBP) superfamily, Endocrin Rev 1999; 20(6):761-87.

43   LeRoith D; Insulin-like growth factor receptors and binding proteins, Clin Endocrinol Metab 1996; 10(1):49-73.

44   Baratta M; Leptin – from a signal of adiposity to a hormonal mediator in peripheral tissues, Med Sci Monit 2002; 8(12):282-92.

45   Guerre-Millo M; Adipose tissue hormones, J Endocrinol Invest 2002; 25(10):855-61.

46   Bjorback C, Hollenberg AN; Leptin and melanocortin signaling in the hypothalamus, Vita Horm 2002; 65:281-311.

47   Playford RJ, et al; Bovine colostrum is a health food supplement which prevents NSAID induced gut damage, Gut 1999; 44:653-8.

48   Playford RJ, et al; Co-administration of the health food supplement, bovine colostrum, reduces the acute non-steroidal anti-inflammatory drug-induced increase in intestinal permeability, Clin Sci 2001; 100:627-33.

49   Bereket A, Lang CH, Wilson TA; Alterations in the growth hormone-insulin-like growth factor axis in insulin dependent diabetes mellitus, Horm Metab Res 1999; 31(2-3): 172-81.

50   Kelly KM, Oh Y, Gargosky SE, Gucev Z, Matsumoto T, Hwa V, Ng L, Simpson DM, Rosenfeld RG; Insulin-like growth factor-binding proteins (IGFBPs) and their regulatory dynamics, Int J Biochem Cell Biol 1996; 28(6): 619-37.

51   Pankov YA; Growth hormone and a partial mediator of its biological action, insulin-like growth factor-1, Biochemistry 1999; 64(1): 1-7.

52   Hosseini S, et al; Colostrum and milk in the treatment of disease, Adv Nutr Res 2001; 10:201-12.

53   Khan Z, et al; Use of the 'neutraceutical' bovine colostrum for the treatment of distal colitis; results from an initial study, Aliment Pharmacol Ther 2002; 16(11):1917-22.

54   Funatogawa K, et al; Use of immunoglobulin enriched bovine colostrum against oral challenge with enterohemorrhagic Escherichia coli O157:h7 in mice, Microbiol Immunol 2002; 46(11):761-6.

55   Huppertz HI, et al; Bovine colostrum ameliorates diarrhea in infection with diarrheagenic Escherichia coli, shiga toxin-producing E. coli and E. coli expressing hemolysin, J Pediat Gastroenterol Nutr 1999; 29(4):452-6.

56   Lissner R, et al; A standard immunoglobulin preparation produced from bovine colostrum shows antibody reactivity and neutralization activity against Shiga-like toxins and EHEC-hemolysin of Esherichia coli O157:h7, Infection 1996; 24(5):378-83.

57   Bitzan MM, et al; Inhibition of Helicobacter pylori and Helicobacter mustelae binding to lipid receptors by bovine colostrum, J Infect Dis 1998; 17(4):955-61.

58   Korhonen H, Syvaoja EL; Bactericidal effect of normal and immune serum, colostrum and milk against Helicobacter pylori, J Appl Bacteriol 1995; 78(6):655-62.

59   Andrew D, Aspinall R; Age-associated thymic atrophy is linked to a decline in IL-7 production, Exp Gerontol 2002; 37(2-3):455-63.

60   Aspinall R, et al; Age-associated changes in thymopoesis, Springer Semin Immunopathol 2002; 24(1): 87-101.

61   Fry TJ, Mackall CL; Current concepts of thymic aging, Springer Semin Immunopathol 2002; 24(1):7-22.

62   Binz K, et al; Repopulation of the atrophied thymus in diabetic rats by insulin-like growth factor-1, Proc Nat Acad Sci 1990; 87(10):3690-4.

63   Burgess W, et al; The immune-endocrine loop during aging: role of growth hormone and insulin-like growth factor-1, Neuroimmunomodulation 1999; 6(1-2):56-68.

64   Clark R, et al; Insulin-like growth factor-1 stimulation of lymphopoesis, J Clin Invest 1993; 92(2):540-8.

65   Geffner M; Effects of growth hormone and insulin-like growth factor-1 on T- and B-lymphocytes and immune function, Acta Pediatr 1997; 423:76-9.

66   Burgess W, Liu Q, Zhou J, Tang Q, Ozawa A, Van Hoy R, Arkins S, Dantzer R, Kelly KW; The immune-endocrine loop during aging: role of growth hormone and insulin-like growth factor-1, Neuroimmunomodulation 1999; 6(1-2): 56-68.

67   He F, et al; Modulation of human humoral immune response through orally administered bovine colostrum, FEMS Immunol & Med Microbiol 2001; 31:93-6.

68   Anwar A, Gaspz JM, Pampallona S, Zahid AA, Sigaud P, Pichard C, Brink M; Effect of congestive heart failure on the insulin-like growth factor-1 system, Am J Cardiol 2002; 90(12): 1402-5.

69   Granata R, Gauna C, Arnolfo E, Atragene D, Broglio F, Ponti R, Ricotti E, Ghigo E; H9c2 cardiac muscle cells express insulin-like growth factor binding protein-3 (IGFBP-3), J Endocrinol Invest 2002 25(S10): 44-6.

70   Li H, Dimayuga P, Yamashita M, Yano J, Fournier M, Lewis M, Cercek B; Arterial
      injury in mice with severe insulin-like growth factor-1 (IGF-1) deficiency, J
      Cardiovasc Pharmacol Ther 2002; 7(4): 227-33.

71   Van Den Beld AW, Bots ML, Janssen JA, Pols HA, Lamberts SW, Grobbee DE;
      Endogenous hormones and carotid atherosclerosis in elderly men, Am J Epidemiol
      2003; 157(1): 25-31.

72   Hosseini S, Inserra P, Araghi-Niknam M, Watson RR; Colostrum and milk in the
      treatment of disease, Adv Nutr Res 2001; 10: 201-12.

73   Spagnoli A, Chiarelli F, Vorwerk P, Boscherini B, Rosenfeld RG; Evaluation of the
      components of insulin-like growth factor (IGF) and IGF binding protein (IGFBP)
      system in adolescents with type 1 diabetes and persistent microalbuminuria:
      relationship with increased excretion of IGFBP-3 18 kD N-terminal fragment, Clin
      Endocrinol 1999; 51(5): 587-96.

74   Thomas F; Increased weight gain, nitrogen retention and muscle protein synthesis
      following treatment of diabetic rats with IGF-1, Biochem J 1991; 276(3): 547-54.

75   Skotiner V; Anabolic and tissue repair functions of recombinant insulin-like growth
      factors, Acta Pediat Scand 1990; 376: S63-6.

76   Steijns JM, van Hooijdonk AC; Occurrence, structure, biochemical properties and
      technological characteristics of lactoferrin, Brit J Nutr 2000; 84(Suppl 1):S11-7.

77   Moddoveanu Z; Antibacterial properties of milk: IgA, peroxidase-lactoferrin
      interactions, Ann NY Acad Sci 1983; 409:848-50.

78   Nord J, Ma P, DiJohn D, Tzipori S, Tacket CO; Treatment with bovine hyperimmune
      colostrum of cryptosporidial diarrhea in AIDS patients, AIDS 1990; 4(6): 581-4.

79   Rump JA, Arndt K, Arnold A, Benedick C, Diehtelmuller H, Franke M, Heim EB,
      Jager H, Kampmann B, Kolb P; Treatment of diarrhea in human immunodeficiency
      virus-infected patients with immunoglobulins from bovine colostrum, Clin Investig
      1992; 70(7): 588-94.

80   Antonio J, et al; The effects of bovine colostrum supplementation on body composition
      and exercise performance in active men and women, Nutrition 2001; 17:243-7.

81   Mero A, et al; Effects of bovine colostrum supplementation on serum IGF-1, IgG,
      hormone and saliva IgA during training, J Appl Pysiol 1997, 83:1144-51.

82   Buckley JD, et al; Bovine colostrum supplementation during endurance running
      training improves recovery, but not performance, J Sci Sport Med 2002; 5(2):65-79.

83   Buckley JD, et al; Oral supplementation with bovine colostrum improves rowing
      performance in elite female rowers. Presented at 5th IOC World Congress on Sport
      Sciences, Sydney 1999 (Abstract: www.ausport.gov.au/fulltext/1999/iocwc/abs246c.htm).

84   Hofman Z, et al; The effect of bovine colostrum supplementation of exercise
      performance in elite field hockey players, J Sport Nutr Exerc Metab 2002;
      12(4):461-9.

85   Kreider RB, et al; Effects of bovine colostrum supplementation in training adaptations
         I: Body composition, Med Sci Sports Exerc 2001; 33(Suppl 5):Abstract LB316.

86   Kerksick C, et al; Effects of bovine colostrum supplementation in training adaptations
         II: Performance, Med Sci Sports Exerc 2001; 33(Suppl 5):Abstract LB317

87   Chan JM, et al; Plasma insulin-like growth factor-1 and prostate cancer risk: a
         prospective study, Science 1998; 279(5350):563-6.

88   Wolk A, et al; Insulin-like growth factor-1 and prostate cancer risk: a population-based,
         case-controlled study, J Nat cancer Inst 1998; 90(12):911-5.

89   Bohlke K, et al; Insulin-like growth factor-1 in relation to premenopausal ductal
         carcinoma in situ of the breast, Epidemiology 1998; 9(5):570-3.

90   Sachdev D, Yee D; The IGF system and breast cancer, Endocrine Related Cancer 2001;
         8:197-209.

91   Ma J, et al; Prospective study of colorectal cancer risk in men and plasma levels of
         insulin-like growth factor (IGF)-1 and IGF-binding protein-3, J Natl Cancer Inst
         1999, 91(7):620-5.

92   How HK, et al; Insulin-like growth factor binding proteins (IGFBPs) and IGFBP-
         related protein-1 levels in cerebrospinal fluid of children with acute lymphoblastic
         leukemia, J Clin Metab 1999; 84(4):1283-7.

93   Sprenger CC, et al; Insulin-like growth factor binding protein-related protein-1
         (IGFBP-rP1) is a potent tumor suppressor protein for prostate cancer, Cancer Res
         1999; 59(10):2370-5.

94   Yang DH, et al; Identification of glycosylated 38-kDa connective tissue growth factor
         (IGFBP related protein 2) and proteolytic fragments in human biological fluids,
         and up-regulation of IGFBP-rP2 expression by TGF-beta in Hs578T human breast
         cancer cells, J Clin Endocrinol Metab 1998; 83(7);2593-6.

95   Yamanaka Y, et al; Characterization of insulin-like growth factor binding protein-3
         (IGFBP-3) binding to human breast cancer cells: kinetics of IGFBP-3 binding and
         identification of receptor binding domains of the IGFBP-3 molecule, Endocrinology
         1999; 140(3):1319-28.

96   Vorweck P, et al; CTFG (IGFBP-rP2) is specifically expressed in malignant
         lymphoblasts of patients with acute lymphoblastic leukemia (ALL), Brit J Cancer
         2000; 83(6):756-60.

97   Travers SH, et al; Insulin-like growth factor binding protein-1 levels are strongly
         associated with insulin sensitivity and obesity in early pubertal children, J Clin
         Endocrinol Metab 1998; 83(6):1935-9.

RESOURCES

Immune-Tree Colostrum6 is laboratory certified as first-milking colostrum obtained within the first six hours of birth, always humanely and from organically raised dairy herds.

www.immunetree.com
877-295-1269

ABOUT THE AUTHOR

DR. ANTHONY KLEINSMITH

Anthony Kleinsmith grew up in the Cache Valley, the heart of Utah's dairy industry, where he learned about the impact of colostrum on survival of newborn calves. He holds a doctorate in nutrition from Chatworth College and a Bachelor of Science degree from the University of Utah. He served as Marketing and Research Director for a prestigious anti-aging health center utilizing growth hormone injections as the basis for anti-aging treatment.

The research he conducted there and elsewhere on growth hormone and first milk convinced him that ultimately the growth and immune factors found in colostrum represented a safer and similarly effective anti-aging effect but with results that could be safely sustained over a lifetime.

Colostrum inspired Dr. Kleinsmith to develop a line of products engineered towards anti-aging, immune enhancement, sports performance and weight loss. These products are now sold in over 40 countries and have been used by over one million people.